PASS OCI (MOCI)
EXAM IN PSYCHIATRY

PASS OCI (MOCI)
EXAM IN PSYCHIATRY

Techniques And Structure You Need

Narinder Panesar
Iveta Valachova

To order additional copies of this book, contact:
Xlibris Corporation
1-800-618-969
www.xlibris.com.au
Orders@xlibris.com.au
500955

Contents

Pass OCI (MOCI) Exam in Psychiatry

Techniques and Structure You Need

Dr Narinder Pal Panesar

MRCPsych, FRANZCP
Consultant Psychiatrist
Mental Health Rehabilitation Unit
Shellharbour Hospital
Shellharbour
NSW

Dr Iveta Valachova

Advanced Trainee in Psychiatry
Braeside Hospital
Sydney
NSW

Preface

It is our great pleasure to introduce this book and share our personal experience of going through one of the most important and challenging exams for admission to the Fellowship of the Royal Australian and New Zealand College of Psychiatrists. The clinical exam tests our ability to present a new clinical scenario in a structured way. This is what we do every day. With repeated presentations and ongoing practice, we have realised that there is a common structure for all cases. On the basis of the constructive and critical feedback from experienced examiners, we were encouraged to reformulate our presentations until we mastered the level expected for the exam. This way, we accumulated material that became the source of this book. We also realised that passing the clinical exam is possible with a positive attitude and a lot of interest in the patient available to us on the day of the exam. It remains true that a psychiatrist can make diagnosis from a patient's history alone, in most of the cases, if he observes and listens to the patient skilfully.

Introduction

Passing the clinical exam for the Fellowship of the Royal Australian and New Zealand College of Psychiatrists (FRANZCP) is one of the most challenging tasks in psychiatry. The exam not only is costly, but also requires significant amount of preparation and commitment. Even good clinicians can fail due to poor techniques. This book aims to provide you with a technique to present cases in a professional and structured way at the clinical exam. It will also help you to revise your existing knowledge. This is the first book written on Observed Clinical Interview (OCI) or Modified Observed Clinical Interview (MOCI) exams. It conveys the authors' personal tips, examples of case formulation, and discussion of the most common exam scenarios and their management. Highlighted is the need to use appropriate questions to obtain adequate history. The book is directed at professionals preparing for the clinical exam in psychiatry. It is also recommended for professionals at all levels of experience who come into contact with psychiatric patients. We hope this small book is a useful contribution to your clinical exam preparation. We would like to thank our examiners for their valuable time and effort in preparing us for the exam.

Dedication

We dedicate this book to our mother Mrs. Satwanti Panesar, who has been our inspiration and moral support.

Acknowledgement

We wish to acknowledge the help and support of Dr Bruce Boman, who prepared us for the clinical exam and reviewed this book.

The Observed Clinical Interview

OCI Exam Structure

- During the Observed Clinical Interview (OCI), you interview a patient for fifty minutes with two examiners observing. The time starts when the patient walks into the examination room.
- Following the time with the patient, you will have twenty minutes thinking time.
- You will then spend time with the examiners, presenting a succinct summary of the salient features, including gaps in the history, mental state examination, a formulation, diagnosis, and differential diagnosis. Examiners then ask you questions.
- In the second part of the exam you present a management plan, and examiners ask questions. The marking has five domains:

I.	Data-gathering process	20 percent
II.	Data-gathering content	20 percent
III.	Mental state examination	20 percent
IV.	Data synthesis	20 percent
V.	Action plan	20 percent

I.　　Data-gathering Process

- The interview process is important as during this time you demonstrate your ability to engage the patient and to obtain relevant information about your patient.
- Suggestion for your introduction to the patient:

'Thank you for coming here today. I am Dr . . . I am a psychiatrist/ psychiatry trainee, and these are my examiners. They will be observing me while I am talking to you. This interview is for the purpose of the exam only, and it will not affect your treatment. It takes forty-five to fifty minutes. What we discuss today is confidential. However, if there is a risk to you or to others, I may need to talk to your treating team'.

- At the beginning of the interview, give the patient a few minutes so that he can talk freely about himself without interruption. During this time, you can reduce your own anxiety and see what your first impression about the patient is.
- It is more important to be attuned to the patient's presentation than giving a list of questions. You can always explain the reasons for not covering all aspects of the history in the gaps.
- Aim for keeping some aspects of the history in your mind without writing everything in your notes.
- Ask only one question at a time.
- During the interview, pick up non-verbal cues, such as changes in the patient's behaviour while he talks about some aspects of the history.
- Aim to do the interview as a challenge and focus on the interaction between you and your patient, without feeling too anxious about the presence of the examiners in the interview room.
- Never give up the interview. It would be a very rare situation that you have to terminate the interview before the allocated time. Unless the patient insists on leaving, ask him to remain in the room till the end of the interview; otherwise you will remember things you wanted to ask as soon as he leaves.

II.   Data-gathering Content

- You must obtain sufficient information about the patient while being empathetic and interested in the patient, and demonstrating active listening.
- Prioritise what areas in the history to cover in depth. Your choice should be guided by the patient's presentation.
- Always demonstrate your knowledge of psychopathology and obtain adequate symptoms to justify your diagnosis and differential diagnosis.
- Demonstrate flexibility of interview style and carefully follow patient clues.
- If a patient gives you important information out of your set interview order, do not interrupt to bring them back, but follow up what they are telling you. You will end up with more useful information that way.

- If you have a suspicion that the patient has a significant cognitive impairment which may impair his or her ability to give a history, aim to do cognitive testing earlier during the interview, e.g. after the initial twenty-five minutes, then complete the rest of the interview.
- Do not assume though that a psychogeriatric patient is cognitively impaired.

The following is a rough guide of the time management during the interview process:

- 0–5 minutes—introduction, explanation, and free talk for the patient
- 5–25 minutes—establish the reason for admission or contact with psychiatric services and clarify symptoms at the time of presentation.
- 25–40 minutes—obtain the past psychiatric history and personal history.
- 40–50 minutes—cognitive testing, limited physical examination, and conclusion of the interview.

III.   Mental State Examination (MSE)

- MSE begins from the moment the patient enters the interview room.
- Focussing on observing the patient with less writing during the interview will give you better understanding of the mental state.
- Always observe for extrapyramidal side effects, akathisia, and tardive dyskinesia. Tardive dyskinesia may become more obvious during cognitive testing.
- Ensure that the MSE correlates with the history, diagnosis, and differential diagnosis.
- Cognitive testing is a part of MSE. In a patient with chronic mental illness, test short-term memory (STM) by asking the patient to register and recall three words; test concentration by asking the patient to name the months of the year backwards (MOYB), and do the frontal lobe tests. If you could not complete cognitive assessment, tell the examiners about it in the gaps, before you present the MSE.

Note: In an elderly patient always aim to complete the MMSE and frontal lobe tests.

IV.   Data Synthesis

Your formulation is perhaps the most important part of your presentation. It tells the examiner you have the skills to be able to put together your history and your observations in a sophisticated way to produce a logical hypothesis. Ensure you have enough time in your twenty minutes thinking time to focus on this task.

The following points are important to include in your presentation:

1. Identifying data
2. Presenting complaints
3. Significant negatives in the presenting complaints
4. Past psychiatric history
5. Negatives in the past psychiatric history
6. Relevant medical, forensic, family, and substance misuse history
7. Functional impairment due to the impact of the long-term illness
8. Risks due to illness and current episode
9. Relevant information obtained from the personal history
10. Gaps
11. MSE
12. Formulation
13. Diagnosis (all V Axes) and differential diagnoses on Axis I.

Your 7–10 minutes presentation and formulation should be well organized and logical.

Essentially you have only 7–10 minutes to offer the examiners your best understanding of the patient. Tell them what you really think about the patient as you do every day.

To provide a sound formulation, offer a list of the most relevant factors in a logical way. Avoid giving details of the history. Initially you can offer your most likely diagnosis followed by your understanding of the factors that lead to the illness. Some guidelines on structuring formulation recommend the use of the headings predisposing, precipitating, and perpetuating factors (the three 'Ps') along the biological, psychological, and social lines.

While formats vary from case to case, the following is an example:

'So in summary, I am presenting a twenty-three-year-old, single, unemployed man on a DSP who was hospitalised two weeks ago with his third manic episode. His phenomenology focuses around an elevated, irritable mood, psychomotor acceleration, and grandiose cognitions. This episode was triggered by the cessation of his maintenance Lithium, heavy stimulant use, and a break-up with his girlfriend.

Vulnerability factors are a genetic loading for bipolar disorder and poor maternal attachment resulting from his mother's depression.

'I would hypothesise that the break-up up with his girlfriend was particularly stressful because of his poor early attachments, leading him to resume stimulant use and stop his Lithium, and then interact with his genetic loading to cause him to become manic.'

The presented information should then be followed by a relevant treatment plan.

V.   Action (Management) Plan

It is good to start your action plan by giving a list of key management issues that you believe are the most important to address in your patient. Then discuss each issue in turn.

The action plan should cover:

- Barriers to the implementation of the treatment
- Evidence to support the treatment
- Likely response to treatment and prognosis
- Role of other professionals
- In a traditional case with a relapse of a chronic mental illness receiving inpatient care, cover the following three stages in approximately equal proportions:
  - i.) Inpatient management (risk management, completion of assessment, and symptom control)
  - ii.) Discharge planning
  - iii.) Ongoing case management and relapse prevention

Other formats will be necessary for a rehabilitation case where you will focus less on acute management and symptom control and much more on improving functioning within the setting of a multidisciplinary rehabilitation team.

Always address carers and family issues.

Although you can have a structure around which you build the management plan, you must prioritise and individualise the management of your patient. The following are the examples:

- When you obtain a collateral history about your patient, tell the examiners what exactly you will ask the GP (e.g. I am calling about Mr X who has lost 10 kg in weight over the last few months. Could you please tell me if he had any investigation done for his weight loss?) or the family (e.g. I will ask his mother what help he offers at home?) and how this will assist you.
- When you adjust a dose of medication, say the exact doses you will use (e.g. I will increase the dose of Venlafaxine XR from 75 mg in the morning to 150 mg in the morning).
- When you discuss the side effects of a medication, say what side effects would be problematic in your patient (e.g. falls in an elderly patient, sedation in a student, weight gain in a female patient).
- If you request or review investigations, say why you want to do them, e.g. LFT in a patient with alcohol problem, ECG prior to commencing Lithium or TCA.
- When you offer psychological therapy to your patient, always say what will be the focus of this intervention (e.g. I will use CBT for depression to challenge his beliefs that he is a burden to his family and shift his cognitive schemas into more positive thinking).
- Demonstrate that you can do the psychological interventions yourself (e.g. family therapy, CBT, or relaxation therapy).
- If you involve an OT, a SW, or a neuropsychologist, always mention why you want them to be involved.
- If you plan to involve the GP for follow-up, clarify what you will ask him (e.g. I will ask the GP to monitor his metabolic profile including weight, BMI, BSL, serum lipids, and blood pressure due to treatment with Olanzapine).

General Tips

- Do what you do every day. Do not introduce new interview techniques for the purpose of the exam. The usual experience is that, when you try to do things differently, you will usually do them badly.
- Try to be relaxed and confident. But do not be arrogant.
- Say, what is your understanding of things happening with your patient.
- Do not attribute features to the patient that he did not demonstrate.
- Do not get into conflict with the examiners.

History Taking

Identifying Data

Acronym: NAMOLS (Name, Age, Marital Status, Occupation, Lives with, Source of referral)

History of Presenting Complaints (HPC)

What happened on the day of admission?

Report symptoms by clusters: (e.g. depressive, anxiety, and psychotic symptoms with examples), their duration, and mode of onset (e.g. sudden or gradual)

Precipitants of the current episode: (e.g. non-adherence/substance misuse/ psychosocial stresses)

Co-morbidity: Anxiety, Depression, OCD, Social anxiety, Panic attacks, Phobias, Substance misuse

Current medications and their side effects

Functioning: impact of the illness on work, social functioning, and relationships

Past Psychiatric History

The first contact with the mental health services: describe the first admission including precipitants, symptoms, and treatment received.

Precipitants of subsequent relapses and admissions: e.g. non-adherence/ substance misuse/psychosocial stresses; pattern of relapses; treatment received in the past including ECT/ depot/ Clozapine/ psychological therapies and their outcomes; awareness of the diagnosis; adherence to medication.

History of deliberate self-harm or suicidal attempts and their triggers.

Pattern of admissions: e.g. self-presentation, brought in by the family or the police

Inter-episodic functioning/Inter-episodic residual symptoms/History of mania in depression/Postnatal Depression in females/Follow-up.

Medical History

Head injury (risk of psychosis/anxiety)/Epilepsy/Diabetes Mellitus/IHD/HTN

Current medical treatment and any change in medication within the last month.

Any known drug allergies.

Family History

Psychiatric illness/ alcohol/ suicide including distant relatives (genetic predisposition).

Forensic History

Conduct Disorder/ ASPD/ AVO/ Imprisonment/ Charges/ Convictions/ Driving under influence/ Violence.

Alcohol/ Drugs/ Smoking/ Benzodiazepines Abuse/ Gambling

Personal History

(For the interview questions please refer to the section on personal history)

Birth and Obstetric Complications

Important in schizophrenia for neurodevelopmental hypothesis and country of origin for migration hypothesis.

Development

Relevant in schizophrenia.

Childhood

Abuse, separation, losses, childhood illness, attachment difficulties →
dysfunctional assumptions of self → schemas or core beliefs formed → triggered
off by critical incidents later in life → reinforces or maintains depression

School/College

Primary/ high/ special schools
Concentration problem (a clue for ADHD)
Dexamphetamine abuse (vulnerability to psychosis)

Occupation

The first employment, the longest job, reasons for changing jobs and the
current source of income.

Relationships

The first relationship, the longest relationship, reasons for break-ups, current
relationship, and sexual preference.

Risks

- Suicide/DSH
- Homicide
- Reputation
- Finances
- Neglect
- Non-adherence
- Driving
- Substance misuse
- Corporate
- Children
- Homelessness
- Disengagement

Functional Decline

Due to the impact of the mental illness (e.g. loss of job, relationship breakdown, social isolation, cognitive decline, and inability to look after themselves).

Gaps

The gaps in the history could be due to a patient being thought disordered, having poor concentration, or due to a complex history.

Elaborate on areas that you would like to explore, e.g. I would like to explore about other psychotic symptoms in details, I would like to complete cognitive testing including frontal lobe tests, I would like to obtain detailed history of polysubstance abuse and dependence, etc.

Questions on Personal History

Many migrants have gone through severe traumatic experiences and it is useful to have a basic knowledge of relevant historical events involving Vietnam, the old Yugoslavia and the Middle East.

Birth and childhood

- Where were you born? (migration hypothesis)
- Was there any problem during your birth that you know of? (obstetric complications)
- Did you have any illness as a child?
- What was your childhood like?
- How many siblings did you have? Where are you in the birth order?
- Tell me about your parents?
- What did your parent do for living?
- How did you get along with your parents?
- How was discipline handled at home?
- Was there any violence at home?
- Did you feel rejected as a child?
- Did anyone ever do something sexual to you that made you feel uncomfortable?
- What is the effect of these experiences on your adult personality?
- Have you experienced losses of loved ones in childhood or later?

- Has your relationship with your parents changed?
- What is your current relationship with your parents?
- What is your current relationship with your child? What would you wish it to be in the future?

School

- Did you enjoy school?
- How did you perform at school?
- Did you go to a special school? (behavioural problems/learning disability)
- Did you have any difficulties in concentrating? (ADHD)
- Did you get into fights? Did you get suspended from school, did you play truant, did you damage property, and were you cruel to animals? (Conduct disorder)
- Were you bullied?
- How did you get along with your teachers?
- How old were you when you left school, did you complete HSC?

Occupation

- What did you do after leaving school?
- How many jobs did you have until now?
- Did you like your jobs?
- What was your longest period of employment?
- How did you get on with your employers and work colleagues?
- When was the last time you worked?
- Were you ever sacked?
- Did you have any friends or did you keep to yourself?

Relationships

- Are you currently in a relationship? For how long have you been in this relationship?
- How is the relationship going?
- How many significant relationships have you had?
- What sort of person are you in relationships?
- Are you in contact with your parents or siblings?
- What do you do in your leisure time?

Mental State Examination

Appearance—Racial origin, Apparent age, Built, Dressed, Unkempt/ Self neglect, Posture, Eye contact, EPSEs (tremor, akathisia, dystonia, Parkinsonism, and tardive dyskinesia), other involuntary movements, gait.

Behaviour—Rapport /Cooperative/ Anxious/ Irritable/ Pleasant/ Psychomotor agitation or retardation

Speech—Spontaneous/Non-spontaneous, Rate (Flow), Volume and Prosody (Tone)

Mood—How patient feels

Affect

- Range of affect
  restricted, blunted (schizophrenia),
  flat (severe depression)
  labile (mania, mixed episode)
- Reactivity
  reactive in normal range (e.g. anxiety, schizophrenia)
  restricted in low range (depression)
  restricted in elevated range (mania/hypomania)
- Congruency
  Congruent/incongruent with mood and thoughts

Thought form (Andreasen N. C. Thought, Language, and Communication Disorders, *Arch. Gen. Psychiatry* 1979; 36:1315–21)

- *Derailment* (includes loosening of associations and flights of ideas)—a pattern of spontaneous speech in which the ideas slip off the track onto another one that is clearly but obliquely related, or onto one that is completely unrelated.
- *Flights of ideas* is a derailment that occurs rapidly in the context of pressured speech.
- *Tangentiality*—replying to questions in an oblique, tangential, or irrelevant manner.

- *Circumstantiality*—a pattern of speech that is very indirect and delayed in reaching its goal idea. The speaker gives many tedious details.
- *Illogicality*—a pattern of speech in which conclusion are reached that do not follow logically.
- *Poverty of thoughts (poverty of content of speech, alogia)*– although replies are long enough so that the speech is adequate in amount, it conveys little information.
- *Poverty of speech (poverty of thoughts, laconic speech)*—replies to questions tend to be brief, concrete, and unelaborated.
- *Incoherence (word salad)*—speech that is essentially incomprehensible at times.
- *Clanging*—a pattern of speech in which sounds rather than meaningful relationships appear to govern word choice (mania, schizophrenia).
- *Neologism*—new word formation.
- *Perseveration*—persistent repetition of words, ideas, or subjects so that once a patient begins a particular subject or a word, he continually returns to it in the process of speaking.
- *Blocking*—interruption of a train of speech before a thought or an idea has been completed.
- *Stilted speech*—speech that has an excessively formal quality.

Thought content

- Includes preoccupation, obsession, overvalued ideas, and delusions
- In depression, assess negative cognitions
  negative view of the world
  thoughts of hopelessness (negative view of future)
  thoughts of worthlessness (negative view of self)
  suicidal ideation or a passive desire to die

Delusions

- *Mood congruent delusion* (in depression)—nihilistic, poverty, guilt, catastrophic (or future disaster), and hypochondriacal (or illness)
- *Mood congruent delusions* (in mania)—grandiose, e.g. belonging to a royal family, being rich, having special talents etc.
- *Mood incongruent delusions* (could be in depression and mania)– persecutory, referential, and bizarre
  Delusions of thought interference (insertion, withdrawal, and broadcasting)

Delusion of control (passivity phenomena)—made actions, feelings, volition (patient says his behaviour is caused by someone else)

- *Somatic passivity* (e.g. patient feels pain in the leg because someone is causing it) versus somatic hallucination (patient feels pain but nobody causes it)

First Rank Symptoms (FRS)

- *Auditory hallucinations*—thought echo, third person, running commentary
- *Passivity phenomena*
  Delusion of thought interference (thought insertion, withdrawal, and broadcasting)
  Delusion of control (made actions, feelings, volition)
- *Delusional perception*
- *Somatic passivity*

Others delusions

Erotomanic, hypochondriacal, persecutory, jealousy, infestation.

These delusions can be symptoms of a delusional disorder or other psychotic illness.

Primary delusions

Delusional perception

Patient gives a delusional meaning to their surroundings for the first time. Primary delusions are usually less common in a full psychotic illness where they are hidden behind secondary delusions.

- Have you had the feeling that something odd is going on that you cannot explain? (*Delusional mood*)
- Did you, at any time, realise that things had a special meaning for you? (*Delusional perception*)

Overvalued idea

A belief held with some doubt or an idea that does not have a delusional intensity.

Obsessional Thoughts or Rituals

Acronym of obsessional thoughts is 'RODSIR' (recurrent, own, distressing, senseless, intrusive, resist)

- Do some thoughts or images keep coming into your mind even though you do not want them to?
- Do you try to resist thinking them?
- Do you have to keep checking or doing activities that you know you have completed?

Depersonalization—Do you ever feel unreal or that part of your body is unreal?
Derealisation—Do you ever feel things around you are unreal? (non specific, can be in psychosis as well as in mood disorder).

Negative symptoms—Affect, Alogia, Avolition, Attention, Anhedonia

Abnormal perception

- *Auditory hallucinations*
  Audible thoughts (patient hears his own thoughts spoken aloud)
  Third person auditory hallucination (e.g. 'he is bad, he is guilty . . . '), running commentary
  Second person auditory hallucinations are usually in depression (e.g. 'kill yourself, you are bad . . . ')
- *Visual hallucinations*—less common in a psychotic illness, more likely indication of an organic brain syndrome, e.g. delirium, dementia.
- *Olfactory hallucinations*—more common in TLE (e.g. patient can smell burning rubber)
- *Tactile/haptic hallucinations*—also in TLE

Cognition

- Orientation in time, place, and person (orientation in person is impaired in severe dementia and dissociation)
- Memory
  Immediate memory and recall, e.g. ask the patient to remember three words
  (e. g 'shirt, brown, honesty') and recall them after a few minutes.
  LTM (long-term memory) e.g. end of the World War II (1945), LTM can be impaired following ECT
- Attention and concentration, ask the patient to spell WORLD backward (DLROW), subtracting serial 7s from 100 (based on MMSE)
  or months of the year backwards (MOYB)—if you do not do MMSE

Frontal lobe testing:

- Clock test
- Similarities and differences, e.g. how are the following two things similar (arm and leg, crying and laughing, sleeping and eating)
- Verbal fluency test (use letter/s 'F'/'A'/'S') a normal test requires at least fifteen words in one minute excluding names of people and places or thirty words in three minutes using all the three letters. Alternatively ask for categories, e.g. animals or supermarket items (a minimum fifteen items required in one minute)
- Set shifting tests—Luria test (fist, edge, palm) or alternating patterns (squares and triangles or 'Go' and 'No Go' test) or Trail making test
- Primitive reflexes (grasp, pout, glabellar tap, palmo-mental)

Insight

1. Insight into having an illness/diagnosis
2. Insight into symptoms/understanding that symptoms are part of the illness
3. Insight into having treatment (What is your attitude towards treatment?)

Judgement is difficult to test and it is usually based on the general content of the interview. Alternatively you can give your patient the following scenario

'Imagine you are standing on one side of a busy road. There are no traffic lights and no pedestrian crossing. How do you get to the other side of the road safely?'

Schizophrenia

The following are suggested interview questions:

Delusion of thought interference

- Are you in control of your thoughts?
- Do you feel that some of your thoughts are not your own?
- Do you think someone puts thoughts inside your head (TI) or takes them out of your head? (TW)
- Do people know what you think about? (TB) or
  Can people read your mind? (TB)
  Do you worry that others may know your secrets? (TB)

Passivity phenomena (actions, feelings, and volition)

- Are you in control of your actions, feelings, and decisions?
- Do you feel someone is controlling them?

Somatic passivity (SP)

- Do you experience any unpleasant sensations in your body? (Somatic hallucination) This should be differentiated from a delusion of somatic passivity by asking the following:
- Are these sensations being caused by someone else or an external force? (SP)

Delusion of persecution

- Are you concerned about your safety?
- Do you worry that others want to harm you?
- Do you think others are watching you, spying on you, following you, or plotting against you?

Delusion of reference

- Does it seem that people talk about you? What do they say? (If the patient can hear what other people say, then it is an auditory hallucination)

- Does it seem that the TV, radio, or newspaper refer to you or give you special messages?
- Do you see any special meaning for yourself in the way things are arranged, e.g. colours, cars, etc?

Delusion of grandeur

- Do you think you have special talents, abilities, or powers?

Delusion of religion

- Do you have a special relationship with God?
- Does he communicate with you in a special way?

Delusions of misidentification

- Do you believe that important people in your life have been replaced by imposters or someone else? (Capgras syndrome)
- Do you believe that strangers are someone who are familiar to you? (Fregoli syndrome)

Delusion of jealousy (Othello Syndrome)

- Does it ever seem to you that your spouse or partner is unfaithful to you?
- What is the evidence for it?
- Have you ever checked their belongings, e.g. a wallet or a diary?
- Have you ever hired a private detective?

Delusion of hypochondriasis

- Are you worried about your body?
- Do you think you have cancer or another serious disease?

Hallucinations

- Do you have unusual experiences of hearing voices when no one is around you or when you are alone?
- Where do these voices come from?
- Do you know them?

- How many voices?
- Are they men or women?
- Do they talk to you (second person) or about you among themselves (third person)? Please give me an example.
- What do they say?
- Do they tell you what to do?
- Do they tell you to hurt yourself or others?
- Do you obey them?
- How do these voices affect your life?

Management of Schizophrenia

A) **Short term:**   i) Safety
                            ii) Completion of assessment or clarification of diagnosis
                            iii) Symptom management
B) **Intermediate term**: Discharge planning
C) **Long term**: Relapse prevention and maximising level of functioning

A) Short term

i   **Safety** (Setting—where to manage the patient/Legal status/Nursing
     observation level)

Risk to self

- Suicide
- Self-neglect
- Reputation
- Non-adherence
- Exploitation (sexual, financial) by others
- Physical health

Risk to others

- Violence (risk factors of violence: young male, substance misuse,
  ASPD, acute psychosis, command hallucinations, delusions of control
  and delusion of persecution)
- Children (risk of abuse, neglect, and domestic violence)

ii   **Completion of assessment or clarifications of diagnosis**

Obtain collateral information from:

- Family (clarify the circumstances of admission, reasons of past
  relapses, pre-morbid, and inter-episodic functioning)
- Review old notes
- Psychiatrist/ Community Case Manager (CCM), (when was the last
  appointment, mental state at the last appointment, past risks, and
  behaviour)
- GP (co-morbid medical illnesses, recent investigations, regular
  medication, and recent changes in medication)
- Liaise with other professionals involved
- Ensure physical examination including waist circumference, height,
  weight for BMI, and EPSEs is completed and organic work-up is
  done.

Investigations:

FBC	Hb (Anaemia) → tiredness can worsen symptoms of mental illness ↑WCC (Infection) → ↓WCC and Neutrophils (Clozapine) ↑MCV (Alcohol abuse) ↑Eosinophils (allergic reaction, Clozapine)
LFT	Liver disease—caution with psychotropic medication ↑GGT (alcohol misuse) Hepatitis B and C (IVD User) Toxic hepatitis (side effect of medication)
EUC and GFR	Dehydration Caution with medication (e.g. Lithium, Amisulpride and Paliperidone are excreted through kidneys)
Drug levels	Lithium, Valproate, Carbamazepine, Clozapine, Nortriptyline
TFT	Relevant in delirium, depression, and dementia
Blood sugar level and Lipid profile	Metabolic screening
Prolactin	For sexual dysfunction, amenorrhoea, infertility, and galactorrhoea
UDS	Drug-induced psychosis
Autoimmune screening	SLE (ESR, Rh Factor, ANA)
Serology	Syphilis (neurosyphilis can present with symptoms of psychosis/mania), HIV
Neuroimaging	CT brain for space-occupying lesion (e.g. Glioma, Astrocytoma) atrophy/ structural changes/CVA MRI brain (allows more precise differentiation between white matter and grey matter); shows lacunar infarct (small infarcts) and demyelination
EEG	TLE, delirium, dementia, CJD, and focal lesions
In elderly	Add serum B12, Folate, CRP to exclude bacterial infection, ECG (for prolonged QTc interval with high dose antipsychotics, critical >500 ms), CXR, MSU.

Rating scales

- BPRS (Brief Psychiatric Rating *Scale)*
- PANSS (Positive and Negative Syndrome Scale*)*
- AIMS (Abnormal Involuntary Movement Scale, 12 items rated 0–4)

iii) Symptom Management

(RANZCP CPG for Schizophrenia 2003)
- Review medication → adjust/titrate dose (give an example)
- D&A → detoxification, relapse prevention
- Treat co-morbidities → liaise with other specialists (e.g. endocrinologist for diabetes mellitus or neurologist for epilepsy)

iv) Psychosocial Interventions (RANZCP CPG for Schizophrenia 2003)

Develop *therapeutic alliance* with your patient, explore patient wishes and expectations

Psychoeducation (NNT 9) increases awareness of illness, symptoms, treatment, and side effects. Evidence shows decreased relapse rates.

Family intervention (FI), (NNT 6.5)

- helps develop an alliance with carers
- reduces emotional distress
- creates positive family atmosphere
- helps problem solving within family
- maintains realistic expectations of patient performance, and
- helps set limits and relationship boundaries

Evidence shows FI reduces relapse rate (>50 percent) and admission rate but does not improve medication adherence.

CBT techniques are being used to improve compliance and psycho-education. CBT is used for treatment of resistant delusions and hallucinations. Evidence shows that it reduces relapse and facilitates recovery and discharge.

Motivational Interview (MI) for drugs and alcohol issues

B) Intermediate term
Discharge planning

- OT—functional assessment, ADLs
- Psychologist—continue CBT
- Social work—accommodation, benefits and financial management, legal issues e.g. guardianship
- Allocation of a CCM
- Family meeting
- MDT meeting

C) Long term
Goals: Relapse prevention and maximising level of functioning

- Early warning signs (EWS) or relapse signature (RS)
- Family Intervention
- Follow-up after discharge
  Review depends on patient's mental state; usually after one week following discharge, fortnightly for one month, then monthly for three months, then quarterly.
  Assess MSE review treatment and side effects.
  Continue monitoring risk.
  CCM—review MSE between appointments, monitor adherence to medication.
- Assertive Community Treatment
- Liaise with D&A team, GP and other specialists where appropriate

- Social Skills Training (SST) is linked with improved functioning.
- Evidence shows that SST improves independent skills, medication and symptom management, social interaction, and communication skills.

- Cognitive Remediation (CR) focuses on improving the following cognitive domains: attention, memory and frontal executive functioning, planning, and decision-making.

- CAT (Cognitive Adaptation Therapy) is used in more severe cognitive dysfunction that impedes learning of living skills. It uses reminders, diary, stickers, and other practical help.

- Vocational Rehabilitation (VR) such as Supported Employment (NNT 4.5) aims to improve economic and social participation. Evidence shows that VR reduces re-hospitalisation and enhances social functioning.

- NGOs (e.g. Schizophrenia Fellowship, SANE—the National Mental Health Charity, ARAFMI)

Bipolar Affective Disorder

DSM IV criteria

Manic episode requires at least one week duration
Hypomanic episode requires at least four days duration
Persistently elevated or irritable mood and at least three of the following:

G P S	DEFG
Grandiosity	Distractibility
Pressure of speech	Excessive involvement in pleasurable activities
Sleep need is decreased	Flight of ideas
	Goal directive activities are increased

Suggested interview questions:

- Have you ever felt so happy as if you were on top of the world? or
- Have you felt so high or irritable that you got into an argument with people? (Mood elevated/irritable)
- During this period have you been overconfident?
- Have you noticed you have special abilities, talents, or powers that others do not have? (Grandiosity)
- During this time, do you talk faster than usual? (Pressure of speech)
- Do you find that your thoughts are racing? (Flight of ideas)
- Do you need less sleep than usual? (Sleep need is decreased)
- Have you been spending more money than you can afford (e.g. shopping)? (Excessive involvement in pleasurable activities)
- Have you noticed an increase in your sex drive? (Excessive involvement in pleasurable activities)
- Have you been doing things that are out of character for you? E.g. driving fast, talking to strangers, or making excessive phone calls? (Excessive involvement in pleasurable activities)

Management of Bipolar Affective Disorder

A) Short term: i) Safety
                        ii) Completion of assessment or clarification of diagnosis
                        iii) Symptoms management
B) Intermediate term: Discharge planning
C) Long term: Relapse prevention and maximising level of functioning

A) Short term

i) Safety (Setting where to manage the patient/Legal status/Nursing observation level)

Risk to self

- Self-harm
- Financial and careless investments
- Sexual promiscuity
- Reputation
- Driving
- Alcohol and drugs

Risk to others

- Violence

ii) Completion of assessment and clarification of diagnosis

Obtain collateral information from:

- Family (What is the patient like when low/high/normal? Inter-episodic functioning? Find out about his behavioural changes when high or low.)
- GP (Co-morbid medical illnesses, e.g. thyroid dysfunction, regular medication, and recent changes in medication)
- Psychiatrist/CCM (When was the last appointment? Mental state at that time and past risks/behaviour when high and low)
- Review old notes

- Liaise with other professionals involved, e.g. neurologist (e.g. for MS), rheumatologist (e.g. for SLE)

Ensure physical examination and organic work-up are done.

If a new presentation

- FBC for anaemia ($\downarrow$Hb), infection ($\uparrow$WBC), alcohol ($\uparrow$MCV)
- LFTs for alcohol ($\uparrow$GGT), hepatitis ($\uparrow$ALT/AST), toxic hepatitis (side effects of medication)
- EUC and GFR for dehydration or for baseline Lithium work-up
- TFTs for primary and pituitary–thyroid dysfunction or drug induced hypothyroidism, e.g. Lithium
- Drug serum levels for Lithium, Carbamazepine, and Valproate
- Autoimmune screening for SLE (ESR, Rh factor, ANA)
- Serology if there is a history of sexual promiscuity—syphilis, HIV (with consent), Hepatitis B and C in intravenous drug users
- UDS
- ECG if commencing treatment with Lithium. Check QTc interval for prolongation, if patient is already on antipsychotics
- Neuroimaging
  - CT scan for SOL/CVA/atrophy
  - MRI for Demyelination/MS
  - EEG for TLE (differential diagnosis)
- CXR, ECG, MSU (always do in elderly)

Rating scales

- YMRA (Young Mania Rating Scale)

iii) Symptom management

(Level of evidence is given in brackets)

Principles

1. Optimise mood stabiliser (increase dose)
2. Switch to another mood stabiliser
3. Combine mood stabilisers
4. Augment mood stabiliser with an antipsychotic (2)
5. ECT (2)

Also treat co-morbidities (e.g. drugs and alcohol abuse, medical conditions)

RANZCP CPG for Bipolar Disorder 2003

Acute mania	Lithium (1), Valproate (1), Carbamazepine (1), Olanzapine (2) Adjunctive treatments: benzodiazepines (5–1) or antipsychotics (5–1)
Mixed episode	Valproate (2), Olanzapine (2), Carbamazepine (4), Lithium (5–1)
Bipolar depression de novo (1st time depression in undiagnosed bipolar disorder)	mood stabiliser: Lithium (1), Lamotrigine (2) or mood stabiliser plus an antidepressant—SSRI/SNRI (2)
Breakthrough depression (onset of depression in established bipolar disorder)	• Optimise mood stabiliser • Add an antidepressant—SSRI/SNRI (2) or • Add a second mood stabiliser: Lithium (1), Lamotrigine (2) • Olanzapine plus Fluoxetine combination • Quetiapine 300–600 mg (not in the college guidelines)
Long-term management of rapid cycling	Valproate (4), Carbamazepine(4), Lamotrigine (4), Lithium (5) If the above treatment fails → Lithium + Valproate
Long-term management of non-rapid cycling	Lithium (1) 0.6–0.8 mmol/L Lamotrigine (2) level not required, usual dose 50–300mg Valproate (2 to 3) 350–700 mmol/L Carbamazepine (2) 17–50 mmol/L

NICE guidelines 2006

1. Treatment of mania or hypomania

Stop antidepressant

Patient *not* on antimanic medication	Patient on antimanic medication
Consider an antipsychotic (if symptoms severe or behaviour disturbed) or	If on antipsychotic—optimize treatment; consider adding Lithium or Valproate
Consider Valproate (avoid in women of childbearing age) or	If on Lithium or Valproate or Carbamazepine—check plasma levels; optimize dose, and/or consider adding antipsychotic
Consider Lithium (if future adherence likely)	
Combine antipsychotic and Valproate or Lithium (if response is inadequate)	

Adjunct therapy (short-term Lorazepam or Clonazepam)

2. Treatment of bipolar depression

- Consider SSRI or Quetiapine in addition to a mood stabiliser
- Switch to Mirtazapine or Venlafaxine
- Add Quetiapine or Olanzapine, if the patient is not already taking them, or
- Add Lithium if the patient is not already taking it.

Mood stabilisers alone are as effective as antidepressant plus mood stabiliser combination (Sachs 2007; Goldberg 2007).

Venlafaxine is more likely to induce a switch to mania (Post 2006; Leverich 2006).

Avoid antidepressants for patients who have either rapid cycling bipolar disorder or a recent hypomanic episode. Instead, consider increasing the dose of the mood stabiliser or adding a second one (including Lamotrigine).

If a patient is in remission from depressive symptoms or symptoms have been significantly less for eight weeks, consider stopping the antidepressant by reducing the dose gradually over several weeks, while maintaining the mood stabiliser.

Consider ECT in people with:

- Severe depressive illness
- A prolonged or severe manic episode
- Catatonia

When using ECT to treat bipolar disorder, consider:

- Stopping or reducing Lithium or benzodiazepines before giving ECT
- Monitoring the length of fits carefully if patient is taking anticonvulsants
- Monitoring mental state for evidence of switching to the opposite pole

3. **Rapid cycling bipolar disorder**

1. Stop antidepressants
2. Evaluate precipitants (thyroid dysfunction, alcohol, medical illness, external stress)
3. Optimise mood stabiliser
4. Consider combining mood stabilisers, e.g. Lithium and Valproate
5. Consider other treatment options, e.g. Aripiprazole, Clozapine, Lamotrigine, Olanzapine, Quetiapine, Risperidone, Thyroxine, Topiramate.

4. **Prophylaxis in Bipolar Disorder**

- Lithium, Olanzapine, Valproate or Quetiapine are first line prophylactic agents
- Treat for at least two years (longer if high risk patients)
- Antidepressant (SSRI) may be used in combination with a mood stabiliser to treat acute episode of depression but should not be routinely used for prophylaxis.
- Chronic or recurrent depression may be treated with an SSRI or CBT in combination with a mood stabiliser or Quetiapine or Lamotrigine.
- Combine Lithium and Valproate for the prophylaxis of rapid cycling.

iv.) *Psychosocial Interventions* *(RANZCP CPG for Bipolar Disorder 2003)*

- Psycho-education (2)
- Family Intervention (2)
- CBT (2)
- Interpersonal social rhythm therapy (IPSRT) (5)
  Lifestyle modification, activities scheduling, regular sleep and meals

B) Intermediate term

Discharge planning

- OT—functional assessment
- Psychologist—continue CBT
- Social work—accommodation, benefits and financial management, legal issues e.g. guardianship
- Allocation of CCM
- Family meeting
- MDT meeting

C) Long term

Goals: Relapse prevention and maximising level of functioning

- Psychoeducation
- Identify early warning signs (EWS)/relapse signature (RS)
- Follow-up after discharge:
  Psychiatrist: after one week, then fortnightly for a month, and then monthly for three months, then quarterly. Review mental state, treatment and side effects, therapeutic levels of medication and adjust treatment, continue risk monitoring.
  CCM: review MSE between appointments, monitor adherence
- CBT
- Family intervention
- Liaise with D&A team, GP and other specialists
- NGOs

Duration of long-term maintenance treatment of Bipolar disorder

- *First manic episode*—continue treatment for *at least six* months from time of recovery
- *Continue long-term maintenance treatment in established bipolar disorder* specified by the following criteria
  - at least two episodes of mania or depression in previous five years, or
  - single manic episode or both hypomanic and depressive episode, or
  - two major episodes of mania and/ or depression irrespective of frequency.

Depression

Always ask about past history of mania

DSM IV features of major depressive episode:

five or more of the following symptoms have been present during the same two-weeks period, at least one of the symptoms is either one or two.

1. Depressed mood
2. Diminished interest (anhedonia)
3. Significant weight loss or a change in appetite
4. Sleep disturbance
5. Psychomotor agitation or retardation
6. Loss of energy or fatigue
7. Worthlessness or excessive guilt
8. Poor concentration
9. Recurrent thoughts of death or suicidal ideation

Melancholic/Endogenous (genetic) Depression

Acronym: DEAD GASP

- Diurnal mood variation (DMV)—worse in the mornings
- Early morning wakening (EMW)
- Anhedonia
- Distinct quality of mood

- Guilt (excessive)
- Appetite or weight loss (significant)
- Suicidal ideation
- Psychomotor retardation or agitation (marked)

Questions:

- How has your mood been most of the time over the past few weeks or months? (persistently low mood)
- Have you noticed that your mood changes over the course of a day? Is it better in the mornings or afternoons? (DMV)

- Do you have problems with falling asleep, staying asleep or waking up too early in the morning? (EMW)
- Have you lost interest in activities that you used to enjoy? (anhedonia)
- Do you feel slowed down? What is your concentration like? (psychomotor retardation)
- Has there been a change in your appetite or taste? Have you lost weight?
- Do you blame yourself for anything? (guilt)
- Do you ever wish not to be alive? (passive desire to die)
- Do you have any thoughts of ending your life? (suicidal ideation)
- Have you made any plans to end your life? (suicidal plans)

Psychotic depression
Mood congruent delusions of

- Guilt
- Nihilism
- Hypochondriacal
- Poverty
- Catastrophic delusion

Questions:

- Have you been feeling guilty or shameful about anything in your life? (guilt)
- Do you believe you deserve punishment? (guilt)
- Do you think other people would be better off without you? (worthlessness)
- Do you think things may improve? Or How do you see your future? *(hopelessness)*
- Do you worry that a part of your body has stopped working or it is dead? (nihilism)
- Do you worry about losing your money or assets, e.g. property? (poverty)
- Do you worry something bad is going to happen to you or your family in the future? (catastrophic)
- Do you worry something is seriously wrong with your health? (hypochondriacal)

Management of Depression

A) Short term: i) safety
                            ii) completion of assessment and clarification of diagnosis,
                            iii) symptom management
B) Intermediate term: Discharge planning
C) Long term: Relapse prevention and maximising level of functioning

A) Short term:

i) Safety (Setting/Legal status/Nursing level of observation)

Risk to self

- suicide
- self-neglect
- physical health, e.g. dehydration, decompensation of diabetes mellitus

Risk to others

- to children, e.g. neglect

ii) Completion of assessment and clarifications of diagnosis

- Family—collateral information about recent behaviour, decline in functioning, suicidal ideation and pre-morbid functioning.
- GP—medication and recent changes in medication, medical co-morbidities
- CCM—ask about engagement, adherence, symptoms, risks, interepisodic functioning
- Psychiatrist—previous contacts including diagnosis and treatment, risks and mental state at the last appointment
- Review old notes for previous diagnosis, treatment received and its effectiveness
- Liaise with other specialists as appropriate

Organic work-up/investigations

- FBC for anaemia or infection (↑WBC)—anaemia can worsen symptoms of depression
- MCV for alcohol use—alcohol is depressogenic
- LFT for alcohol (↑GGT), hepatitis (↑ALT/AST)
- EUC and GFR for Lithium work-up or dehydration
- TFTs for primary and pituitary–thyroid dysfunction or drug induced hypothyroidism, e.g. Lithium
- Autoimmune screening for SLE (ESR, Rh factor, ANA)
- B12/Folate/Vitamin D—deficiency can worsen symptoms of depression
- ECG prior to starting TCA or Lithium (to exclude arrhythmias)
- UDS for drug use especially cannabis or amphetamine—withdrawal can cause depression
- Brain CT scan/MRI scan for CVA, vascular depression, white matter hyperintensities, MS, TBI
- CXR and MSU (in elderly)—physical illness can cause/worsen depression

Rating scales

- BDI (Back Depression Inventory) self-rated
- HAMD (Hamilton Rating Scale for Depression)
- MADRAS (Montgomery-Asberg Depression Rating Scale)
- GDS (Geriatric Depression Scale) self-reported

iii) Symptom Management

RANZCP CPG for Depression 2004 (Level of evidence is given in brackets)

1st line	
Mild Depression	Lifestyle change and problem solving(2)
Moderate depression and Dysthymia	SSRI / CBT/IPT (1)
Severe uncomplicated depression	TCA /Venlafaxine /CBT/IPT(1)

Severe complicated depression (melancholic/ psychotic depression)	TCA/SNRI-Venlafaxine(1), Duloxetine or Desvenlafaxine (not in the college guidelines)
Atypical depression	Phenelzine/CBT/IPT (1)

If no response:

2nd line		
If on SSRI	change to	Venlafaxine (SNRI)/TCA(1)
If on Venlafaxine/SNRI/TCA	then	↑ dose add CBT/IPT(1)
If Atypical depression (on Phenelzine)	then	Add CBT/IPT(1)
If no response to the above	then	Augment with Lithium(1) levels 0.4–0.6 (for augmentation)/ Atypical antipsychotic/T3/ high dose Venlafaxine (5)
If no response to the above	then	ECT

CBT plus antidepressant give better results than either treatment alone for depression or for co-morbid anxiety and depression.

ECT is the most effective treatment for Treatment Resistant Depression (TRD).

TMS (Transcranial magnetic stimulation) has not been accepted as an effective treatment for TRD

UK NICE Guidelines 2009

- Mild depression—antidepressants are not recommended; use guided self-help, CBT, or exercise.
- Moderate to severe depression and dysthymia—SSRI
- Severe depression—antidepressant plus CBT
- TRD—augment with Lithium, antipsychotic, or a second antidepressant.
- Severe and TRD—use ECT.

Maintenance treatment for Depression

- In psychotic depression, aim to discontinue antipsychotic three months after full remission.
- Maintenance dose of antidepressant is the same as the response dose
- Maintenance treatment is for one year for the 1st episode and three years for recurrent episodes

Pharmacological Management of TRD (literature review)

1. **Augmentation of an antidepressant with**

   - *Lithium* (Crossley and Bauer, 2007) meta-analysis; augmentation with Lithium was significantly more effective than placebo, 40 percent of participants on Lithium responded in comparison with 17 percent on placebo.

   - *T3*—Prange et al. 1969, studied T3 mainly with TCA (Imipramine). Data on T3 augmentation to SSRIs from recent randomized trials are not as convincing as for TCA (Current Opinion in Psychiatry, 2007, 22: 7–12)

   - *Atypical antipsychotics* (Papakodas et al. 2007) meta-analysis of augmentation with atypical antipsychotics in TRD—significantly more effective than placebo (J Clin psychiatry, 2007, 68:826–832)

   - *Pindolol*– Ballesterol, Callado 2004, meta-analysis of augmentation of SSRI with Pindolol showed that Pindolol is not effective in TRD. Geretsegger 2008, Paroxetine with Pindolol, double blind RCT also failed to demonstrate efficacy of Pindolol in TRD.

2. **Change of antidepressant**

STAR-D (Can J Psychiatry 2010)

There is no difference in effectiveness between treatment with antidepressants and the levels of treatment. Every new trial of treatment increases a chance of recovery from depression.

3. **Addition of a second antidepressant or commencement of a combination of two antidepressants**

- *SSRI plus TCA* (Fava 2001; Nelson 2003) open studies—a combination was more effective than either alone. Monitor risk of cardiotoxicity (ECG).
  Citalopram and Sertraline are safe as they do not have significant P450 activity.

MAOI, the most effective antidepressants in melancholic and non-melancholic TRD (Parker 2001) and in TRD non-responsive to TCA (Nolen 1993). Avoid combinations: Tranylcypromine with stimulants (risk of hypertensive crisis), and TCA with MAOI

Address co-morbidities

- Consult with D&A team
- Liaise with appropriate medical specialists

iv.) Psychological Interventions

Develop therapeutic alliance

- Psychoeducation
- Family intervention
- CBT (based on your understanding of the patient, give a few examples how you will implement CBT strategies in this patient)
- Interpersonal psychotherapy (IPT)

Social

- Accommodation
- Finances
- Legal issues

B. Intermediate term

Discharge planning

- OT for functional assessment
- Psychologist for continuation of CBT
- SW to address accommodation, benefits, and financial or legal issues, e.g. guardianship
- Allocation of CCM
- Family meeting
- MDT meeting

C. Long term

- Follow-up after discharge from hospital: after a week, fortnightly for a month, then monthly for three months, then quarterly
- Involve CCM to monitor mental state, adherence to medication, and offer support
- Psychiatrist to review mental state, risks, response to medication and their side effects
- Psychoeducation—ongoing
- Family intervention
- CBT/IPT
- Liaise with GP and other specialists
- Treat co-morbidities including liaising with D&A team
- Consider NGOs support

Anxiety Disorders

Generalised Anxiety Disorder (GAD)

Uncontrollability of worries distinguishes GAD from normal worries.

DSM IV criteria:

Symptoms persist for *at least six months* most days than not.
At least three of the following symptoms:

Acronym: **TRICS** Fatigue

- Tense muscles—reflection of fight and flight response that prepares the body for fight
- Restlessness
- Irritability
- Concentration problem
- Sleep problems (initial ± middle insomnia)
- Fatigue

Questions:

- Are you a worrier? or Would you say you are an anxious person?
- What do you worry about?
- Do you think your worries are excessive (unrealistic)?
- Do you have physical symptoms with your worries like tense muscles, palpitation, abdominal distress, chest discomfort, or headaches?
- How do your worries affect your life (work, relationships, functioning)?

Management of GAD

CBT is the treatment of choice (TOC) 12–16 weekly sessions.

Pychoeducation as a component of CBT

- Explain the nature of anxiety as response to stress that prepares the body for fight and flight response
- Explain associated somatic symptoms of anxiety (tension in muscles, tremor, sweating, fast breathing, racing heart and urinary frequency)
- Reassure the above symptoms are *not* dangerous and to certain extent they are normal in stress. But when these symptoms become severe, anxiety becomes counterproductive and it requires treatment.

Be aware of the following cognitive patterns in GAD

- Intolerance of uncertainty and overestimation of risk and cost are the core features of anxiety
- Worries about future, catastrophic outlook, search for certainty, emotion-focused rather than problem-focused approach to worries, reassurance-seeking behaviour are other cognitive patterns of GAD.
- Beliefs about benefits of worries such as 'If I worry, it will not happen', or 'If I worry enough, I will be able to find a solution'. Such beliefs can relieve anxiety in a short time but make GAD persist.
- Anxiety provoking situations are avoided and hence never mastered.
- Anxious person has a tendency to interpret ambiguous cues as threatening.

Behavioural strategies

- Breathing exercise (explain how to practice it as if you were explaining to your patient)
- Progressive muscle relaxation (explain how to practice it)
- Lifestyle modification, e.g. regular exercise
- Distraction, yoga, meditation
- Mindfulness based task-focused activities
- Sleep hygiene (provide details)
- Challenge patient's beliefs with behavioural experiments
- Gradual exposure to the avoided situations (give examples how to implement it to your patient)

Cognitive strategies

- Cognitive strategies are aimed at modification of cognitive errors about anxiety.
- Explain that intolerance of anxiety and overestimate of threats are the core features of GAD.
- Explain that avoidance of anxiety-provoking situations, beliefs in benefits of worries and reassurance seeking maintain GAD.
- Ask patient to monitor episode of worries and their triggers.
- Redirect your patient towards mindfulness based on focusing on task at hand.
- Instruct patient to resist urges to engage in worries, instead suggest focus on task at hand.
- Instruct your patient to repeat this approach as often as necessary, even every few minutes.
- Teach your patient how to use problem-focused strategies instead of emotion-focused solution to worries.
- Discuss a realistic estimate of threats, and identify a likelihood that patient's worries become reality.
- Encourage your patient to tolerate uncertainty and doubts.
- Ask your patient to practice exposure to uncertainty through tolerating doubtful thoughts and images without seeking reassurance.

Pharmacological treatment (NICE guidelines 2007)

If possible, avoid benzodiazepines, as they reduce effectiveness of CBT and cause rebound anxiety. Benzodiazepines should not be used beyond 2–4 weeks.

Benzodiazepines have advantage for somatic symptoms of GAD
Antidepressants have advantage for cognitive symptoms of GAD

- 1st line treatment:
    - SSRIs—start small dose (half of the recommended dose), initially it may worsen symptoms through side effects
    - Mirtazapine/Venlafaxine/Duloxetine
- 2nd line treatment:
    - TCAs (Imipramine/Clomipramine)
    - β-blockers (Propranolol)
- Other treatments: Quetiapine 150 mg daily (not included in NICE guidelines)

Panic Disorder and Agoraphobia

Always check suicidality in Panic Disorder

DSM IV criteria for Panic Disorder:

1. Recurrent unexpected panic attacks
2. At least one of the attacks has been followed by one month (or more) of one of the following:
    a. concerns about having another attack
    b. worries about the implications of the attack or its consequences (e.g. having a heart attack, losing control)
    c. change in behaviour related to the attacks

DSM IV criteria for Panic Attack:

A period of an intense discomfort with at least four of the following:

(Autonomic)

1. palpitations
2. sweating
3. shaking

(Chest and abdomen)

4. shortness of breath
5. feeling of choking
6. chest pain or discomfort
7. nausea or abdominal distress

(Psychological)

8. dizziness
9. de-realization or de-personalization
10. fear of losing control
11. fear of dying

(General)

12. numbness or tingling sensation
13. chills or hot flushes

Questions:

- Have you ever had a panic attack?
- Can you describe the panic attack?
- What happened to your body during the panic attack? (shakes, sweating, shortness of breath, fast heart rate, butterflies in your stomach, hot and cold flushes, tingling around mouth and in fingers, dizziness and fear of going crazy or dying or losing control)
- How often and how many?
- Do you fear having another attack?
- Does anything bring them on (if yes, specific phobia)?
- Do they occur in specific situations? E.g. social situation—social phobia; or in places from where an escape would be difficult—agoraphobia
- Do you worry being in crowded places, travelling on public transport, driving a car, being away from home alone? (agoraphobia)
- Do you avoid these situations?
- Does having someone with you help? (agoraphobia)
- Are you uncomfortable in social situations? (social phobia)
- How uncomfortable do you get? Do you get to the point of having a panic attack? (social phobia)
- Do you avoid social situations? (social phobia)
- Do you worry about speaking, writing, and eating in front of people? (social phobia)
- Do you worry about embarrassing yourself? (social phobia)

Management of Panic Disorders (RANZCP CPG 2003)

CBT is the TOC (NNT 3) versus Medication (NNT 6)

Psychological treatment

- Psychoeducation
- Explain the cause of a panic attack in a simple way, e.g. that a false trigger from the brain to the body causes a panic attack.
- Reassure that symptoms of panic attacks are *not* dangerous.
- Explain that the patient can learn how to control the symptoms of panic attacks.

Behavioural (relaxation) strategies

- Teach breathing exercise (explain how to practice it as if you were explaining to your patient)
- Progressive muscle relaxation (explain how to practice it)
- Graded exposure (for avoidance behaviour) based on hierarchy situations that your patient has identified. Patient can begin with imaginary exposure followed by hierarchy situations.
- Lifestyle modification, e.g. regular exercise.

Cognitive strategies

- Modification of cognitive errors about anxiety.

Pharmacological Treatment

Avoid benzodiazepines

- 1st line treatment: SSRIs (starting with a small dose); explain the possibility of initial worsening of symptoms due to side effects.
- 2nd line treatment: Mirtazapine

Evidence for

- CBT
    - less dropout rate
    - longer relapse prevention at two year follow-up

- TCAs
    - Efficacy equal to CBT
    - ↑ dropout rate due to side effects
    - ↑ relapse on discontinuation (30 percent)

- Benzodiazepines
    - Less effective than TCAs
    - fewer dropout rate due to less side effects
    - ↑ relapse rate on discontinuation

- SSRIs
    - modestly effective
    - less dropout rate
    - ↑ relapse rate on discontinuation than CBT

- Combination of CBT plus medication is not better than either alone.

- Treatment with benzodiazepines is associated with poor outcome.

Post Traumatic Stress Disorder (PTSD)

Acute—   Duration of symptoms less than three months

Chronic—   Duration of symptoms more than three months

With delayed onset—   Onset after six months

Acronym: DREAMS

Disinterest, detachment, and numbness
Reliving of the event in nightmares and flashbacks
Extreme nature of a traumatic event
Avoidance of situations which are reminders of the event
Months—duration of the disturbance is more than a month
Sympathetic overarousal with exaggerated startle response

Questions:

- Have you experienced any significant trauma in your life? What sort of experience was it? (Extreme event)
- Do you have a lot of bad memories of the trauma?
- Do you have nightmares/flashbacks of this experience?
- Do you feel that you are reliving the event in your nightmares or flashbacks? (Re-living)
- Do you avoid situations that remind you of the event? (Avoidance)
- Since the event, have you lost interest in things you used to enjoy? (Disinterest)
- Since the event do you feel emotionally numb? (Numbness/ Detachment)
- Do you feel edgy all the time/startle easily (e.g. difficulties in sleep, concentration and irritability)? (Sympathetic overarousal)
- How has this trauma affected your life?

Management of PTSD

Psychological therapy is the TOC

CBT (12–16 weekly sessions)

- Education about the nature of PTSD
- Self-monitoring of symptoms
- Anxiety management
- Graded systemic desensitisation (exposure)
- Relaxation and breathing exercises
- Cognitive restructuring

EMDR (Eye Movement Desensitisation Reprocessing)

- It is a CBT technique that uses hand/finger to induce horizontal eye movements.
- Patient focuses on finger movements for 10–15 minutes.
- EMDR activates traumatic memories that the patient cannot recall or experience in a normal state.
- The recalled memories are accompanied by emotions.
- The patient then gains relief (in presence of the therapist in the safe environment)

Pharmacological treatment

(The Maudsley Prescribing Guidelines, 10th Edition)
Do not offer pharmacological treatment as a routine first-line treatment.
Use hypnotic medication for sleep disturbance only for short term (2–4 weeks).

- 1st line treatment: SSRIs (can also help co-morbidities)
- 2nd line: Mirtazapine/TCAs(Clomipramine)/Venlafaxine/augmentation with antipsychotics
- Treatment Resistance: Phenelzine

When an adult PTSD sufferer responds to drug treatment, continue the treatment for at least twelve months before gradual withdrawal (NICE guidelines, 2005).

Obsessive Compulsive Disorder (OCD)

Experiencing anxiety due to obsessions and relief from anxiety after compulsions is typical of OCD.

Obsessions

- Are you an obsessive person? Have you ever had unpleasant thoughts or images that kept coming into your head and were difficult to stop or to get rid of?
- Do some thoughts or images keep coming into your mind even though you do not want them to? (acronym: RODSIR—Recurrent, Own, Distressing, Senseless, Intrusive, Resist)
  Are they your own thoughts (OCD) or do they come from an outside source? (Psychosis, thought insertion)
- Do you try to resist them? What is the reason behind your obsessions? E.g. fear of contamination, doubts etc.

Compulsions

- Do you do things over and over again, e.g. checking locks, turning the stove off, or washing your hands?
- What would happen if you did not do these things?
- Once you have done it (e.g. checking and washing), do you feel it is completed or not?
- How much time in a day do you spend on these things?
- How have they affected your life?
- Do you find yourself counting things?
- Do you get intrusive sexual images?

Management of OCD

Exposure Response Prevention (ERP) is the TOC.
Cognitive therapy—no proven benefit.

ERP (each session can last between forty-five minutes to two hours)

- Educate about anxiety, e.g. explain that symptoms initially peak, then subside.
- Reassure that anxiety is *not* dangerous and it is treatable.
- Explain how treatment works, re-experiencing anxiety through a graded exposure to more difficult tasks (as per hierarchy of compulsive behaviours).
- Create a hierarchy of difficult situations which produce compulsive behaviours.
- Ensure patient does not use other mental activities, e.g. counting to compensate for the original compulsions.
- Ask your patient to practice the achieved hierarchy task at home.
- Involve family members in understanding the treatment to enable them to avoid reassurance.

Pharmacological treatment

(The Maudsley Prescribing Guidelines, 10th Edition)

- 1st line treatment: SSRIs/Clomipramine
- Augmentation with antipsychotics
- Others: A combination of pharmacotherapy plus psychological treatment may be the most effective treatment.

Eating Disorders (ED)

Anorexia Nervosa (AN)

- Restricting types
- Purging types

DSM IV features

1. Body weight <85 percent of that expected
2. Intense fear of gaining weight or becoming fat.
3. Body image disturbance in the way in which one's body weight or shape is experienced.
4. Amenorrhoea: the absence of at least three consecutive menstrual cycles in post-menarcheal females.

Questions:

- Have you ever had concerns about your body weight? Or Are you concerned about your weight?
- What is your current weight and height (Weight/M^2=BMI)
- What is your ideal weight? Are you afraid of gaining weight?

Food

- Have you ever dieted?
- Have you ever restricted certain foods like fats, sugars, or carbohydrates?
- What do you eat on a normal day? What did you eat yesterday (breakfast, lunch, dinner, and snacks)?

Exercise/purging

- Are you doing anything to achieve your ideal weight, e.g. dieting, exercise, purging (laxatives, diuretics, vomiting)?

Amenorrhoea and medical problems

- What about your periods? When was your last period?
- Do you have any medical problems such as dizziness, palpitation, and tiredness?

Eating Disorder Not Otherwise Specified (EDNOS) is the commonest ED and it is always a differential diagnosis.

Bulimia Nervosa (BN)

- Purging type
- Non-purging type

DSM IV criteria:

1. Recurrent episodes of binge eating
    -   eating in a discrete period of time, e.g. within any two-hour period
    -   a sense of lack of control over eating during the episode
2. Recurrent inappropriate compensatory behaviour in order to prevent weight gain (self induced vomiting, misuse of laxatives, diuretics, enemas or other medications, fasting and excessive exercise)
3. 1 and 2 occur, on average, at least twice a week for three months
4. Self-evaluation is unduly influenced by body shape and weight

Questions:

- Do you ever have binging episodes when you eat a large amount of food in a short period of time?
- What all do you eat during a binge?
- Do you feel out of control when you binge?
- How do you feel after a binge?
- What do you do to prevent weight gain?
  Do you purge? (vomiting, laxatives, diuretics)
  Do you exercise?
- Do you worry about gaining weight?
  What is your current weight?
  What do you think about it?

- What about your periods?
- Do you have any medical problems after you purge?

Rule out co-morbid depression/OCD/D&A/BPD

Management of AN, BN, and EDNOS

- Due to overlap of symptoms between AN and BN, the approach has much in common. This approach will also apply to EDNOS, the most common category of ED. We will refer to the management of ED, unless stated otherwise.
- Confirm diagnosis and exclude co-morbidity, e.g. depression, OCD or substance misuse, particularly stimulants and alcohol.
- Liaise with GP to exclude organic causes of weight loss such as hyperthyroidism, diabetes mellitus, and Crohn's disease. With the patient's permission, obtain collateral information about the onset of the problem and family situation. Find out if there are other children or members in the family with similar problems.
- *Physical examination:* Look for evidence of weight loss and cachexia, anaemia, lanugo body hair, hypotension, bradycardia, hypothermia, loss of muscle mass and prominent bones, swelling of parotid and submandibular glands, eroded tooth enamel and Russell sign if purging. Patients with AN are often reluctant to seek treatment. Patient with BN are more likely to engage in treatment but resist recommendations.
- Treatment of ED involves a multidisciplinary team approach (psychiatrist, psychologist, physician/ endocrinologist, dietician, nurse).
- The aim of treatment is to restore weight in AN and to restore normal eating pattern in BN. Treatment starts with establishing a good therapeutic relationship and engagement in a program that includes psychoeducation, individual and group CBT, family therapy, medical management, and monitoring.
- *Psychological treatment* is the TOC. It involves family intervention, if the patient is still supported by family. CBT and problem solving is more suitable for those living independently. CBT involves psychoeducation and cognitive restructuring of automatic negative thoughts related to eating behaviour, food, attitudes about weight and body shape. It

offers helpful techniques on how to manage binges, e.g. by delaying a binge or using a chewing gum. It also involves homework for monitoring behaviour, cognitions, and feelings about eating and related problems.

- Family intervention includes education about ED, understanding how family behaviour contributes to the disorder, reassurance that family is not the cause of the ED, improving communication within the family, and using positive reinforcement (rewards) for weight gain.

- *Pharmacological treatment:* Medication should not be offered as a sole treatment for AN. Medication can be used for co-morbid conditions such as depression; however depression may resolve with the restoration of weight. Due to patient's medical complications of low weight and purging such as electrolyte imbalance, there is an increased risk of side effects and the dose of medication should be reduced. Patients with AN should be supplemented with Thiamine as there is a risk of re-feeding syndrome.

- Fluoxetine has been shown to be effective in reducing binges in the treatment of BN.

- *Restoration of normal eating pattern:* Depending on the severity of the ED, gradual restoration of eating behaviour can be achieved in the day hospital with meal supervision or as an inpatient. Patients are encouraged to eat three meals per day, eat in a company of others, and retain meal after eating by avoiding purging behaviour or exercise. Unhealthy beliefs about eating are gradually restructured through CBT (e.g. using laxatives does not mean weight loss, eating regular meals does not mean weight gain, etc).

- *Physical treatment:* Please see the conditions requiring an inpatient treatment in the table below.

Guidelines for inpatient admission (RANZCP CPG for Anorexia Nervosa 2004)

Medical status	HR <40 min, BP <90/60 mm, low potassium, other electrolyte imbalance, temp <97°F(36.1°C); orthostatic changes: >20 bpm increase HR; >20 mm drop in BP
Suicidality	An active plan
Weight	BMI <14
Anorexic cognitions	Continuous preoccupation, cooperative only in highly structured treatment
Co-morbidity	Other psychiatric disorder requiring hospitalization
Eating	Needs supervision of every meal, nasogastric tube feeding
Exercise	Needs reminding to restrain and/or modify
Purging and vomiting	Compulsive, uncontrolled activity
Environment	Severe family problems
Treatment availability	Requires residential placement

HR, heart rate; BP, blood pressure.

- If your patient is severely underweight and dehydrated, the aim of treatment is to rehydrate, stabilise weight, and correct any electrolyte imbalance. Regular monitoring of electrolytes (Na, K, Cl, Ca, P, Mg) and ECG (prolonged QTc, bradycardia) is essential.
- A target weight should be discussed in collaboration with the patient. Aim for an average weekly weight gain of 0.5 kg in outpatient setting and 0.5–1 kg in inpatient setting (NICE, 2004).
- NGT (Nasogastric tube) may need to be considered if patient keeps losing weight during the inpatient admission.
- Involve dietician to provide advice on gradual increase of calorie intake to avoid re-feeding syndrome.
- During the inpatient admission or at the day program, staff offers support during meal times, monitor food intake, and monitor any attempt to hide food or perform other activities such as exercise to lose weight.

Alcohol

DSM IV criteria:

A maladaptive pattern of substance misuse leading to clinically significant impairment or distress that is manifested by 3 or more of the following, occurring at any time in the same twelve month period:

1. Tolerance
2. Withdrawal
3. Use of alcohol in larger amounts or over a longer period
4. Persistent desire or unsuccessful efforts to cut down or control use
5. Great deal of time is spent in activities necessary to obtain alcohol
6. Neglect of alternative activities (social, occupational, or recreational) because of alcohol
7. Use is continued despite knowledge of having physical or psychological harm

CAGE ≥ 2 → 95 percent chance of abuse/dependence

Questions:

- Have you ever felt that you should **C**ut down on your drinking?
- Have you ever been **A**nnoyed when people criticised your drinking?
- Have you ever felt **G**uilty about your drinking?
- Have you ever needed to take a drink first thing in the morning to steady your nerves (**E**ye-opener) or to get rid of a hangover?

Present

- When did you drink last?
- What did you drink (wine, beer, sprit)?
- How often do you drink? Find pattern (binge/abuse/dependence)
- Describe a typical day for me?
- Have you noticed that you need more drink to get the same effect? (Tolerance)
- What happens if you did not have a drink or cut down for a few days?(Withdrawal, nausea, vomiting, shakes, sweating, anxiety,

agitation, headache, disorientation, hallucinations, visual, tactile, auditory, fits, blackouts/delirium tremens)
- Do you crave for a drink? (Craving)
- Do you find it difficult to control drinking? (Difficult to control)
- Did you try to cut down or stop but could not?(Persistence)
- Do you neglect your health, family, work, and hobbies due to alcohol? (Neglect)
- Do you find alcohol is the most important part of your life? (Primacy)

Past

- When did you start drinking?
- When did you start drinking regularly?
- When did you first notice alcohol as a problem?
- Have you ever been abstinent from alcohol? For how long?
- What made you restart drinking alcohol?
- How did you maintain abstinence?
- Did you take medication or see a psychologist or attend alcoholics anonymous (AA)?

Consequences

- How has alcohol affected your life in terms of health (gastritis, hepatitis, pancreatitis, hypertension and cardiomyopathy) work, family/ relationships, MVA/TBI?
- Have you ever been convicted of drunk driving or had trouble with the law?

Calculations

1 unit (1/2 pint) = 8–10 gm alcohol

Recommended number of units: men 21 units/week and women14 units/week

Simple formula to calculate number of units consumed per day:

Number of units = volume in litres × percentage of drink
For e.g. 375 ml (1 can) of beer (0.375 litre) × 3.5 percent = 1.3 units of alcohol

Number of units of common drinks

Beer mid-strength (3.5%)	1 can	1unit
Beer full-strength (4.8%)	1 can	1.4 units
Wine 11.5%-13%	1 glass (100ml) 1 bottle (750ml)	1 unit 8 units
Spirits 40%	1standard measure(30ml) 1 bottle (700ml)	1 unit 22 units

- What change did you notice in your mood during an abstinence of ≥4 weeks? (temporal relationship between alcohol and depression).
- Did your mood (or anxiety) improve during abstinence? Improvement in mood is expected if low mood or depression was due to alcohol use.

Management of Alcohol Withdrawal

Assess severity of alcohol use. Alcohol Withdrawal Scale (AWS) has seven items.

1. Perspiration 0–4
2. Tremor 0–3
3. Anxiety 0–4
4. Agitation 0–4
5. Axilla temperature 0–4
6. Hallucinations 0–4
7. Orientation 0–4
   Severity of alcohol is based on ASW sore

Mild	1–4
Moderate	5–9
Severe	10–14
Very Severe	15+

A medical review is required if AWS is >10

Pharmacological treatment

- Diazepam is the treatment of choice (caution in liver dysfunction, COPD, cardiac failure) for alcohol withdrawal or detoxification.
- Use Oxazepam in liver disease (Diazepam 5mg = Oxazepam 15mg)
- Use haloperidol for delirium tremens
- Thiamine 100 mg I/M daily for three days, then once daily orally for prophylaxis of Wernicke's encephalopathy.

Borderline Personality Disorder (BPD)

Acronym: BIAS IRA

- Are you an emotional person? Does your mood swing rapidly from being happy to being sad in a matter of minutes or hours? (Affect instability)
  Will symptoms change in response to environmental events within hours?
  (e.g. Dysphoria in the context of a troubled relationship. A threat of abandonment is due to borderline dynamics versus dysphoria with hopelessness occurs in a depressive disorder)
- What sort of person are you in relationships? (Relationship)
  Are you sensitive to rejection?
  Do your relationships with friends tend to be intense with ups and downs?
- Do you harm yourself, if something goes wrong in your life? What did you do in the past? (Self-harm)
- Do you often feel empty in yourself? (Boredom)
- Are you an impulsive person? Has that ever gotten you into trouble like drugs, sex, reckless driving, spending, binge eating)? (Impulsive)
- Do you have difficulties in controlling your anger? (Anger)
- Do you bottle it up or let others know that you are angry?
- What do you do when you are angry?
- Do you sometimes feel that you don't know who you are? (Identity)

  - BPD has unstable affect fluctuating between irritability and depression
  - BPD has a feeling of inner badness and loneliness
  - Melancholic features are rare in BPD
  - Dysthymia is common
  - BPD is not a variant of unipolar depression
  - Treatment of depression does not result in remission of BPD
  - Bipolar disorder is more common in families of BPD
  - 11–23 percent of patients with BAD II met criteria for BPD (Paris et al.)
  - Presence of BPD and other personality disorders were robust predictors of accelerated relapse after remission from depressive episode

Management of BPD

Psychological treatment is the TOC

Dialectical Behavioural Therapy (DBT):

- DBT combines individual and group therapy
- DBT is not effective for depression in BPD
- DBT is effective in patients with suicidal and self-harming behaviour
- DBT is for patients who are very chaotic and without structure

DBT aims to address four main areas:

1. Reduce suicidal and self-harm behaviour
2. Therapy interfering behaviour
3. Quality of life interfering behaviour—to reduce frequent hospitalisation, interpersonal problems, and drugs and alcohol problems
4. Enhance specific skills to cope more effectively

DBT has four modules:

1. Mindfulness skills—central to DBT
2. Interpersonal effective skills—how to deal with interpersonal conflicts
3. Emotional regulation skills—understanding emotions and how to reduce emotional vulnerability
4. Distress tolerance skills—how to tolerate distress and accept life as it is

Mentalisation Based Therapy (MBT)

MBT has effect on both depression and BPD and it is as efficacious as DBT. The principles of MBT can be used in everyday practice. The principles of MBT have lot in common with Gubderson's 'good enough' treatment for BPD. The therapy will help them reflect on their own state of mind which they usually inhibited because of early trauma or abuse. The therapist validates their distress. MBT is focused on the quality of relationship with the patient.

Gubderson's 'good enough' treatment principles:

- Weekly individual sessions
- Active collaboration with patient
- Psychoeducation
- Validation, empathy, active, and curious approach
- Negative transference is actively addressed
- Reflection is encouraged
- Here and now focused
- Building a narrative—'able to make a sense of yourself and your life'
- No explicit focus on self-harm behaviour
- No explicit skill training
- Wise use of medication
- Outcomes similar to DBT

Psychiatric Formulation

The formulation is a synthesis of data that links the patient's history with findings on mental state examination which results in making a putative diagnosis. The most important aspect of a good formulation is your understanding of the patient as a person during the interview. Based on the quality of data you have gathered during the interview process along with your ability to make connections between different aspects of the history, the formulation is generated. The table below provides some examples of different aspects of the history in guiding you to build the formulation, when you are interviewing a patient.

Factors→ ↓	Biological	Psychological	Sociocultural
Precipitants/ current stressors	Substance abuse, medical illness, non-adherence to treatment	Adverse life events, losses, separation, divorce, anniversaries	homelessness, isolation, financial losses
Predisposing/ vulnerability	Genetic vulnerability, low IQ; developmental delay, head injury, drug abuse	Personality, sexual abuse, early losses and traumas, loss of parents, low self-esteem, unresolved grief	Domestic violence, unemployment, disrupted family, financial hardship
Perpetuating	Non-adherence to treatment, resistance to treatment, substance abuse	Personality, poor coping skills, lack of role model, low self—esteem, temperament	poor support, family dynamics, isolation, unemployment, high expressed emotions
Protective/ Strengths	No substance abuse, good response to medication	Good pre-morbid functioning, good insight	Family support, religion

Make sure you understand the longitudinal picture of the illness, not only the most recent episode. Always ask about the first episode and its precipitants as the pattern of the illness is often repeated in the future episodes. Furthermore, the course of a chronic illness brings significant functional changes in patient's life. You are expected to identify these changes and their causes as perpetuating factors.

Always start with identifying data and what is wrong with the patient. If you are unsure of the diagnosis, give a summary of clinical symptoms and features of mental state suggestive of a diagnosis.

Do not only give a list of relevant predisposing, precipitating, and perpetuating factors without linking them together and explaining how these factors affects the patient's presentation. In the formulation, demonstrate that you have capacity to provide at least one link between the patient's past history and current presentation. Following are the examples to make the link between the past and present. All are cognitive models except the Attachment theory.

- Early experiences of abuse have contributed to later abusive or aggressive behaviour via *'identification with the aggressor'*, depression through problems with guilt/ self-blame and low self-esteem, and relationship failure through problems with trust.
- Early attachment problems can lead to difficulty forming or sustaining relationships later in life
- Long stay in hospital during early childhood can lead to difficulties forming secure attachment
- Insecure attachment in childhood predisposes to depression, anxiety, and emotional instability in later life
- Early experiences of physical illness can predispose to later dependency or somatisation
- Conflict with an authority (parent) in childhood can lead to problems with compliance and medical advice
- Early losses (e.g. loss of parent <11 years) predispose to depression
- Overprotective/controlling parents make children vulnerable to depression, anxiety, eating disorder, and dependency
- Problematic relationship with parents leads to higher rates of depression in early adolescence

- Early environmental factors (insecure attachment, late childhood traumas) predispose to BPD, early onset dysthymic disorders and depression
- Attachment difficulties lead to poor self-esteem and lack of skills to buffer stressors ending in depression
- Postnatal depression has effect on the relationship where infant and child's subsequent development is mediated by maternal attachment style, which can predispose to depression and anxiety

You can also use stages of cognitive development formulated by Erik Erikson in your formulation. The most commonly used stages are:

- Role confusion (13–20 years): relevant in formulating early onset of schizophrenia.
- Stagnation (40–60 years): the occupational and personal failures in middle age can lead to depression.
- Despair (age 60+): decline in physical health or dissatisfaction with past life can lead to anxiety and depression in elderly.

Erikson's eight stages of psychosocial development

Stages	Age	Development	Basic strengths
Infancy	0 to 18 months	Trust vs. Mistrust	Drive and Hope
Early childhood	18 months to 3 years	Autonomy vs. Shame	Self control, Courage, Will
Play age	3 to 5 years	Initiative vs. Guilt	Purpose
School age	6 to 12 years	Industry vs. Inferiority	Method, Competence
Adolescence	12 to 20 years	Identity vs. Role confusion	Devotion, Fidelity
Young Adulthood	20 to 40 years	Intimacy vs. Isolation	Affiliation, Love
Middle Adulthood	40 to 60 years	Generativity vs. Stagnation	Production, Care
Late Adulthood	Over 60 years	Integrity vs. Despair	Wisdom

Case Examples

The following examples are brief presentations of salient features, MSE, formulation, differential diagnoses, and management.

Case example 1: Schizophrenia, paranoid type

(ID)

Mr C.S. is a twenty-eight-year-old man of Asian background living with his mother and two younger siblings on disability support pension for schizophrenia, currently being looked after by his mother.

(PC)

Mr C.S. was brought to the hospital by his sister after having a fight with strangers in a local suburb in response to psychotic experiences. He experienced *persecutory delusions* as he believed that strangers wanted to harm him; he had *delusions of reference* from car number plates to fight and kill his persecutors. In addition, he experienced *command hallucinations* instructing him to harm others, and *third person auditory hallucinations* talking about him. He had sleep and appetite disturbances but no suicidal ideation or negative cognitions. He felt sad and attributed this feeling to his beliefs.

(HPC)

Several weeks prior to the admission, he was non-adherent to Clozapine 400 mg daily and used approximately 1gm of cannabis daily. At the same time his mother was diagnosed with a recurrence of bowel cancer.

(PPH)

Of note is a history of poly-substance abuse between age sixteen and twenty-one. Mr C.S. was using mainly THC, but also speed, ice, and heroin. He denied intravenous drug use. It is not known whether he had psychotic experiences during this time. Based on the assessment, it is likely that he was dependent on substances and he supported his habit by drug dealing. However, I have no details about symptoms of tolerance, withdrawal, or adverse impact of substances on his physical health supporting this assumption.

I understand that he had developed his initial psychotic experiences when age twenty-one. This was a stressful time in his life when his mother had her first bowel cancer surgery. At that time, he cut his arm in response to psychotic symptoms. Furthermore, he got involved in conflicts with strangers and was taken to a police cell, and then transferred to a local hospital. He was initially managed with different antipsychotics, prior to treatment with Clozapine. He responded to Clozapine, but he did not reach remission. His had two previous hospital admissions due to non-adherence to Clozapine and substance misuse.

(Negative history)

There was no history of negative symptoms of schizophrenia, no history of depressive, manic and PTSD symptoms. He denied significant medical and family history. He also denied forensic history.

(Functional impact of mental illness)

Due to ongoing persecutory and referential delusions, he leads a socially isolated lifestyle, mostly staying at home and doing house chores. His illness causes not only social isolation but also puts him at a risk of aggression towards those that he recognises as his persecutors.

(Significant personal history)

Mr C.S. was born overseas. Of significance are numerous losses throughout his life especially in his home country. He left for Australia as an illegal refugee when he was nine years old, after his father was killed in his home country. After many difficulties, he was granted a visa and brought his family from overseas. Consequently, he started using substances. Throughout the early years of his childhood and adolescence, he missed on family relationships, upbringing, social skills, and education. Of note are the similarities between persecutions his family suffered overseas and his persecutory delusions.

(Gaps)

The gaps in Mr C.S.'s history are due to the complexity of his past experiences. I would like to know more details about his past and current substance use and dependence, and how this affected his mental and physical health. I would also like to know more about his personal life, his relationship with his mother, siblings, and social network.

Mental State Examination

Mr C.S. presented himself as a young man of Asian background. He was clean but unkempt and unconcerned about his appearance. He was wearing a blue polo shirt and dark brown pants. He had no extrapyramidal side effects, TD or akathisia.

He was cooperative, with good rapport and eye contact.

His speech was normal in rate, volume, and prosody.

His affect was restricted in low range, thought, and mood congruent.

There was no formal thought disorder. He reported delusions of reference and persecutory delusions.

He experienced third person and command auditory hallucinations.

He was oriented to time, place, and person.

He demonstrated normal testing in frontal domains. He scored 3/5 on MOYB and 2/3 on STM.

Formulation

Mr. C.S. is a twenty-eight-year-old single man of Asian background, on DSP with a history of paranoid schizophrenia over the last seven years. He was admitted to hospital due to a relapse of chronic psychotic illness in the context of non-compliance with Clozapine at the time of increased stress because of the fear of losing his mother to bowel cancer. In addition he was abusing cannabis.

He has no known genetic vulnerability to a mental illness. He experienced several significant losses and life traumas including migration. His illness was precipitated by substance use during a time of significant stress, when he feared loss of his mother who had bowel cancer surgery. He separated from his family when he was only nine years old and missed on the development of the Erikson's stage of industry. The lack of psychosocial development, a lack of identity, as well as an ongoing use of substances make him vulnerable to stress. A fear of the loss of his mother as the main supportive figure would mean another separation and thus has a significant impact on his mental state. Thus, he developed another psychotic episode at the time of a perceived separation from his mother, when she had a relapse of bowel cancer.

Differential Diagnosis

Axis I:

1. Schizophrenia, paranoid type.
2. Schizoaffective disorder: Requires a combination of symptoms of a mood disorder and schizophrenia, but psychotic symptoms must be present for at least two weeks in the absence of mood symptoms. His presentation did not satisfy these criteria.
3. Poly-substance abuse

Axis II: Defer
Axis III: No medical illness
Axis IV: Unemployment, social isolation
Axis V: GAF 30–40 (His behaviour is considerably influenced by delusion and he has major impairment in functioning)

Management

Short-term management

Inpatient treatment will focus on symptom management and establishing therapeutic relationship.

I will maintain his confidentiality, unless there is a risk involved.

I will obtain collateral history about his functioning at home and precipitants of his aggression. I will ask details about substance use, e.g. amount of each substance he used in the past, duration of use, symptoms of withdrawal and an impact of substances on his physical health including hepatitis C and HIV. Further questions will focus on his interpersonal relationships. I will contact his GP to find out about his physical health including hepatitis C. I will also speak to his community team to find out his engagement with the services in the past. I will review UDS and organic work-up to exclude any medical illness and side effects of treatment with Clozapine (neutropenia, myocarditis, cardiomyopathy, blood sugar level, and serum lipids). I will be interested in his weight gain, metabolic profile including waist circumference and other side effects more commonly associated with Clozapine such as sedation and salivation.

I will administer AIMS test to identify motor side effects of a long-term antipsychotic use. I will review his past medications and side effects and review his current treatment. Clozapine will be the most suitable choice, if he can comply with treatment. If his symptoms persist after optimizing Clozapine dose, I will consider Clozapine augmentation with other medication for example, Amisulpride or Risperidone.

Early in the treatment, I will provide psychoeducation about his illness and the importance of compliance with Clozapine.

I will assess his readiness for change and use the Motivational Interview to minimise substance use.

I will assess his suitability for CBT focused on his delusional beliefs, compliance and motivation.

I will contact his mother and siblings and address their concerns. I will provide ongoing psychoeducation to them. I will also aim to minimise high expressed emotions (EE) and provide carer's support.

Discharge planning

Discharge planning starts at the early stage of admission through involvement of multidisciplinary team, community services, and the family.

With help of an occupational therapist, I would like to know his level of functioning and his suitability for a future vocational rehabilitation. I will involve his CCM in discharge planning and formulating a patient-focused care plan.

With the help of a social worker, I would like to know about his financial needs.

Long-term management

Post discharge follow-up will focus on relapse prevention and maximising his level of functioning.

I would like to review him regularly following discharge; the first appointment within a week of discharge. If he is on Clozapine, I will liaise with the clozapine clinic for follow-up as per Clozapine protocol.

I will discuss the importance of minimising stress and maintaining a regular sleep pattern and a healthy lifestyle. I will explain that sleep disturbance is a common symptom which heralds another psychotic episode.

As a strategy for relapse prevention, we will discuss about the 'early warning signs' of relapse through the exploration of symptoms that he could use to indicate a further episode of psychosis.

Other strategies focussed on improving his functioning include CBT for long-standing delusions, Motivational Interview techniques for maintaining abstinence from substances, and family intervention for sustaining suitable family environment and preventing relapse.

Case example 2: Major Depression in elderly

(ID)

I saw Mrs Jo, a seventy-one-year-old married mother of four adult children, who lives alone. Mrs Jo was admitted to the hospital due to a suicidal attempt in the context of a depressive episode.

(HPC)

Mrs. Jo had cut her wrist prior to the admission. On assessment, she presented with low mood, insomnia, loss of appetite and weight loss, decreased activities, and thoughts of worthlessness. She experienced *mood congruent nihilistic delusions* that her whole body, particularly her bowel, was not working. She experienced *delusions of guilt* as she inappropriately blamed herself for telling lies to doctors. She also experienced mood *incongruent persecutory delusions* that someone was watching her and wanting to harm her to get rid of her; and *referential delusions* that people were talking about her. In addition, she reported *audible thoughts* ('follow me'). She also reported *anxiety symptoms,* and *panic attacks* (episodes of breathlessness, chest pain, shakiness, and dizziness). She did not remember what medication she was taking. Her complaints worsened over a period of few months. There was no psychosocial precipitant. This was her first presentation to mental health services.

(Negative PPH)

Mrs. Jo had no past psychiatric history including PND or mania. There was no history of DSH and no family history of mental illness. There was no reported history of substance abuse or forensic history.

(Medical history)

Of note is her medical history of hypothyroidism, supplemented with Thyroxine, pulmonary fibrosis on long term Prednisone, hypertension on antihypertensive medication, and obesity.

(Functional impact of the illness)

Her depression impacted her level of functioning with reduction in activities, self-neglect, and weight loss. She also had difficulties with memory and concentration that could increase the likelihood of further cognitive decline in the future.

(Risks due to illness)

Due to her depressive and psychotic symptoms, she was at risk of disorganised behaviour, non-compliance with medical treatment, deterioration of her physical health, and self-harm.

(Relevant personal history)

Mrs. Jo presented as a resilient person who grew up in an environment of domestic violence. Her parents separated when she was eight years old. At twelve, she lost her mother to cancer. Consequently, she lived with her aunt's family and she disliked her uncle. When she was sixteen years old, she left for Tasmania where she worked in a factory and got married. She described her marital life as unhappy. Her father, with whom she had only limited contact, died a year ago.

(Gaps)

The gaps are related to her difficulties with concentration throughout the interview.

I would like to know more about her current treatment, available support and her functional decline at home. I would also like to complete cognitive testing including frontal testing.

Mental State Examination

Mrs. Jo presented as an elderly lady, initially guarded but warmed up during the interview. She was clean but unkempt and unconcerned about her appearance. She was wearing a warm jumper and brown pants appropriate to the weather. She looked tired. She was alert and maintained good eye contact.

Her speech was reduced in rate and volume.

Her affect was restricted in depressed range. Her mood and thoughts were congruent with affect.

There was no formal thought disorder.

She reported mood congruent and incongruent delusions and audible thoughts. She also experienced thoughts of worthlessness. She denied further suicidal ideation or a desire to die.

She scored 21/30 on MMSE (concentration 1/5; recall 1/3; verbal comprehension 1/3; orientation to time 4/5, wrong date).

Her insight was partial as she was aware of feeling depressed, but she perceived her psychotic symptoms as reality not as symptoms of her illness. She accepted treatment.

Formulation

Mrs Jo is a seventy-one-year-old married lady admitted to the hospital due to a suicidal attempt in the context of a depressive episode with psychotic features. Her medical co-morbidities are important factors in triggering this episode, especially long-term treatment with Prednisone, possible thyroid dysfunction, and anti-hypertensive medication. The significant factors predisposing her to depression are her early loses such as the death of her mother when age twelve and a lack of a nurturing figure, conflicting relationships with men in her life, and finally a loss of her father prior to this admission. In addition, she had been dealing with deteriorating physical health. She was stagnated in the Erikson's stage of despair.

Differential Diagnosis

Axis I

1. Major depressive episode with psychotic features
2. Major depressive episode due to thyroid dysfunction, Prednisone and anti-hypertensive treatment

   3.   Schizoaffective disorder
   4.   Cognitive disorder NOS (dementia versus pseudodementia)

Axis II Defer
Axis III Thyroid dysfunction, hypertension, pulmonary fibrosis
Axis IV Social isolation, loneliness
Axis V GAF 30–40

Management

Short-term management

Short-term management will focus on safety, symptom management, and treatment of medical co-morbidities.

Ensuring her safety will be a priority. I will monitor her suicidal ideation and treat her depression.

I will review her old medical notes, looking for her past treatment of thyroid dysfunction. I will also be interested in her recent brain CT looking for vascular changes and brain atrophy. I will obtain collateral history from the family and her GP about her pre-morbid functioning.

Early in the treatment, I will educate her about depression, its treatment, and side effects to improve her insight.

I will review her oral intake and hydration. I will review her current thyroid function, and other medical co-morbidities that could contribute to her discomfort, e.g. UTI. Due to a history of medical co-morbidities, I will liaise with her endocrinologist and respiratory physician to understand the severity of her illness.

I will review her current antidepressants and antipsychotic medication and their side effects, e.g. hyponatremia. However, as I am not aware of her current treatment, I will consider her on Escitalopram 10 mg in the morning and Risperidone 0.5 mg in the evening as initial doses.

With her permission, I will contact her family, organise a family meeting, and involve them in her care and support.

I will assess her suitability for CBT or IPT focusing on the late life issues such as losses, grief, decline in functioning, and coping with medical illness.

I will repeat MMSE and frontal lobe testing after remission of depression to differentiate between pseudo-dementia and dementia. Depending on the result, I will consider neuropsychological testing.

I will involve a SW and an OT to assess her level of functioning and independence at home and services required following her discharge.

If compliance becomes an issue, I will consider using a Webster pack.

I will provide her with emergency contact details prior to the discharge.

Long-term management:

Long-term management will focus on maintenance of remission and providing community support.

I will continue regular reviews in the community and communication with her family, until her care can be transferred back to her GP. During these reviews, I will identify her complaints including depressive symptoms, physical difficulties, and psychosocial stresses.

I will communicate with her GP and other specialists and ask them to review her physical health.

I will review her pharmacological treatment including side effects. As this is her first episode of depression, I will aim to continue antidepressant treatment for a year; antipsychotics should be gradually discontinued, a few months after remission.

I will aim to continue CBT or IPT (e.g. to improve her coping skills to cope with her ill health).

I will continue monitoring cognition to identify early dementia and consider neuropsychological assessment.

I will aim for involving her in increased social activities.

I will also consider a referral to age care services for assessment of appropriate support at home (e.g. cleaning, shopping, outing).

Case example 3: Consultation Liaison case

(ID)

Mrs. C.L. is a fifty-nine-year-old mother of three adults, living with her husband, managing her own take away restaurant and caring for her elderly father.

(PC)

She was admitted to hospital for worsening of depression since her last discharge from the same hospital three weeks ago. On admission, she presented with diurnal mood variation, anhedonia, lack of energy, initial insomnia, self-neglect, memory problems, critical view of self, and thoughts of worthlessness. She denied suicidal ideation but reported a passive desire to die. She also had so called 'mini-seizures'; symptoms suggestive of panic attacks but these were difficult to differentiate from epileptic fits and/or dissociative states.

(PPH)

She has a past history of depression that started during her first marriage and a suspected episode of PND. She reported recurrent depressive episodes over the last three years. A year ago, she had an episode of mania after her last surgery for pituitary adenoma. During the manic episode, she experienced elevated mood with reduced sleep and appetite and denied concerns about having pituitary adenoma.

(Negative PPH)

There is no history of OCD, substance use, family history of mental illness or forensic history.

(Medical history)

She has a medical history of pituitary adenoma and she is on replacement therapy, with Hydrocortisone and Thyroxin. She had two surgical interventions; the last surgery was a year ago. She also has a history of restless leg syndrome.

(Functional impact of illness)

Her illness impacted on her functioning with increased social isolation, self-neglect, and changes in her personality. In addition, when she was manic, she crashed her car and lost her driver's licence. This puts her at a risk of self-harm and reputation.

(Relevant personal history)

Mrs. C.L. was born in a large metropolitan city. She had a close relationship with her mother who had memory loss due to Alzheimer's dementia in late age. She had difficulties with her primary education due to impaired hearing. When she was ten, her parents separated and she was close to her stepfather. At age seventeen she became a single mother. After her boyfriend left her, she attempted suicide by poisoning. There were no further suicidal attempts. Her first marriage was to a man from a different religious and cultural background with traumatic experiences. They had three children. She remarried and her husband is supportive.

(Gaps)

The gaps in the history were due to her impaired concentration. I would like to complete cognitive testing including MMSE and frontal lobe testing. I would also like to clarify her episodes of 'mini-seizures' particularly to rule out epilepsy. Furthermore, I would like to find out about her past history of depression and treatment.

Mental State Examination

Mrs. CL presented as a pleasant, engaging and cooperative Caucasian lady with obvious psychomotor retardation, looking older than fifty-nine years. She maintained good eye contact.

She had no make-up. She was casually dressed and clean but not concerned about her appearance.

Her speech was normal in rate, volume, and prosody. Her mood was low.

Her affect was restricted in low range and congruent with her mood.

There was no formal thought disorder, no mood congruent and incongruent delusions, and no suicidal or homicidal ideation. However, she reported a passive desire to die. She was preoccupied with negative cognitions and thoughts of worthlessness.

Her cognition was impaired throughout the interview. She required questions to be repeated. Frontal lobe testing was impaired. Due to time restrictions, I was unable to complete MMSE.

She had insight about her depression but not about mania.

Formulation

Mrs. C.L. is a fifty-nine-year-old business owner and a carer of her elderly father, presenting with a depressive episode on the background history of a bipolar affective disorder characterised by recurrent episodes of depression and a manic episode. She also experiences episodes of 'mini seizures' that require further clarification.

She is predisposed to an affective illness due to past traumatic experiences such as the divorce of parents, teenage pregnancy, and abusive first marriage.

Her current episode of depression was most likely precipitated by hormonal changes associated with pituitary dysfunction.

In addition, her serious health problems are accompanied by memory loss possibly due to central hypothyroidism. She fears memory loss that reminds her of her mother with Alzheimer's dementia. Furthermore, she grieves the loss of her own personality due to medical and mental health problems. She is stagnated at the Erikson's stage of despair.

Differential Diagnosis

Axis I:

1. Bipolar Affective Disorder, current episode depressive due to hormonal changes and pituitary adenoma.
2. Adjustment disorder with depressed mood

Axis II: Defer
Axis III: Pituitary adenoma with hormonal dysfunction
Axis IV: Carer's stress/ functional decline
Axis V: GAF 40–50 (serious symptoms and serious impairment in functioning)

Management

Short-term management

Her treatment will require effective communication among different specialists including an endocrinologist, a neurologist, a neurosurgeon, and her GP.

I will ensure her safety in the ward by regular reviews and monitoring of her mental state.

I will complete her assessment and with her consent, I will obtain collateral history from the family, GP, and the endocrinologist for better understanding of association between her mood and hormonal treatment. I will review her progress notes and discuss her history with the previous treating team.

I will find out about changes from her pre-morbid functioning as a result of pituitary adenoma.

I will review her current investigations, including brain MRI, TFT, cortisol level, prolactin, EUC, LFT, FBC, B12, Folate, EEG, ECG, CXR, and MSU.

I will review and adjust current medication doses, if required. However, as I am not aware of her current treatment, the most appropriate approach would be to treat her for a bipolar depression with a mood stabiliser (e.g. Sodium Valproate 500 mg twice daily as a starting dose) and if necessary, an antidepressant (e.g. Escitalopram 10 mg in the morning).

I will liaise with the neurologist to exclude epilepsy and the endocrinologist for supplementation of pituitary gland.

With her permission, I will engage her family in her care. I will provide her psychoeducation to increase her insight.

Once she recovers from depression, I will repeat her cognitive screening test and consider a neuropsychological assessment.

I will consider her for CBT for negative cognitions, when her concentration improves. Due to a change of role and a grief for her loss of personality, she may be benefit from IPT.

Discharge planning

I will involve an OT for functional assessment.

I will also involve a SW for financial assistance and introduce a CCM.

Long-term management

I will focus on a relapse-prevention through identifying early warning signs, using psychoeducation and life style modification. I will monitor her mental state, compliance with medication, and their side effects at the outpatient clinic. I will review the serum levels of Sodium Valproate quarterly.

I will communicate with her GP and other specialists.

I will continue CBT and problem-solving techniques to improve her coping skills following discharge.

I will provide carer's support and liaise with a local geriatric team to consider a respite for her elderly father, while she is recovering from a depressive episode.

I will provide her with emergency contacts of the crisis team.

Case example 4: Late onset Schizophrenia

(ID)

Lisa is a sixty-two-year old Philippine widow, mother of one adult daughter, living alone. She was admitted to the hospital due to her daughter's concerns about her declining functioning. She presented with a two-year history of untreated psychosis.

(PC)

The main presenting problem was a fear for her safety due to psychotic symptoms. Lisa believed that her neighbour wants get her out of her unit to be able to grow cannabis. She reported *referential delusions* about his behaviours such as making loud noises, slamming doors, pacing up and down in front of her door, hitting the wall and throwing stones at the kitchen walls. She stated the purpose of this behaviour was to intimidate her. She experienced second person *auditory hallucinations* such as hearing her neighbour swearing at her, calling her names, and threatening to kill her. Furthermore, she experienced sleep and appetite problems, and anhedonia. Lisa's dysphoria was almost as disabling as her psychotic experiences. She had vague suicidal ideation but no plans. She had affective symptoms but not a major depressive episode, her delusions were mood incongruent. She did not know what treatment she was getting in the hospital.

(HPC)

Lisa gives a history of well systematized delusional beliefs about her neighbour over the last two years. During this time, she has had persistent psychotic symptoms. The onset of her illness was preceded by significant events in her life two years ago. These included the diagnosis and surgery of bowel cancer, followed by chemotherapy and its side effects. In addition, she developed a pulmonary embolism and rectal bleeding while on warfarin. She was aware of the significance of her medical condition and the gravity of the situation. After she returned home from hospital, she first started experiencing psychotic symptoms. Since then, she has not been free of psychotic symptoms. The significance of her illness was related to her husband dying of bowel cancer a year earlier.

She does not have a history of negative symptoms of schizophrenia, previous psychiatric history, or a history of self-harm. In the past, she saw a counsellor due to conflict with her daughter who ran away from home. There is no family history of a mental illness and no drug and alcohol history.

(Functional impact of illness)

Lisa's illness has been associated with declining social functioning and suicidal ideas in the context of frustration with her psychotic experiences. Her fears have restricted her life inside her unit as well as outside. As a consequence of these fears, she has stopped cooking in her unit, going to the balcony, or going out.

(Relevant personal history)

In contrast to her current mental state, Lisa is a resilient lady with good pre-morbid functioning, in spite of her limited educational background. Lisa functioned well in her home country. She has raised her daughter as a single mother, coped with migration stress, and the responsibilities of caring for her sick husband, who subsequently died from bowel cancer. She exhibited strong resilience and coping strategies, up until she developed cancer.

Lisa was born into a poor family to a single mother as the middle of five children, grew up in a rural area of Philippines but had a good relationship with her siblings. Keen on social life, she ran away from home to seek a better future for herself. She became a mother in her adolescence, but her boyfriend left her just as her father left the family. Prior to migrating to Australia, she coped as a single mother with the extensive support of her family. She married an older man living in Australia, seeking a better future for herself and her daughter. She worked throughout her life in Australia up until she became a carer for her sick husband. A very stressful life event was when her daughter left home.

(Gaps)

The gaps in the history are numerous, especially psychopathology, specifically psychotic and affective symptoms, including mania.

Mental State Examination

Lisa presents as a young, short, and slim Philippine female. She was casually dressed and clean, without concerns about fashion.

Lisa was pleasant and cooperative, maintaining reasonable eye contact. There was no psychomotor retardation or psychomotor agitation, and no EPSE, akathisia or tardive dyskinesia.

Her speech was accented, at times difficult to understand, normal in volume, with preserved prosody. She spoke spontaneously and her speech was not pressured.

Her mood was sad and less scared than before.

Her affect was restricted in low range as a result of her psychotic experiences. She was tearful during the interview, but there was some reactivity.

Her thought form was circumstantial.

Lisa was preoccupied with psychotic symptoms as reported earlier. She reported suicidal ideation but no plans. She denied homicidal thoughts, particularly towards her neighbour.

She had no insight into her mental illness, symptoms, or treatment.

Her cognition was consistent with the level of her education.

Formulation

Lisa is a sixty-two-year-old widow living alone, on an aged pension with a two year history of paranoid schizophrenia. This is her first presentation with declining functioning and fears due to preoccupation about psychotic symptoms.

The illness was precipitated by a series of events, diagnosis, and surgery of bowel cancer, chemotherapy and its side effects, significant haemorrhage, and pulmonary embolism.

She was vulnerable to develop an illness due to fear of death related to her husband's death from bowel cancer. She had looked after her husband who died of bowel cancer, she developed bowel cancer and it frightened her. Social isolation and lack of care from her daughter reinforced this fear. Lisa sacrificed her life for her daughter who did not meet her needs when she developed major health problems. Complications and medical co-morbidities further confronted her with her own mortality.

Lisa developed this psychotic episode at the time of social isolation, and under the influence of significant stressors from the physical illness.

Differential Diagnosis

Axis I:

1. Late onset schizophrenia
2. Schizoaffective disorder (if she had co-morbid mood symptoms)
3. Psychotic disorder due to bowel cancer
4. Major depression due to bowel cancer
5. Major depression with psychotic features

Axis II: Defer as there was no indication of a personality disorder; she was a resilient person
Axis III: Bowel cancer in remission, history of PE, and rectal haemorrhage while on Warfarin
Axis IV: Social isolation, conflict with the neighbour
Axis V: GAF 40–50 (serious symptoms and serious impairment in functioning)

Management

Short-term management

The aim of the treatment is to reduce her distress from her symptoms and provide social support that she has been lacking.

I will complete assessment and with her consent I will obtain collateral history from her daughter and GP focusing on pre-morbid functioning and medical co-morbidities.

I will review her organic work-up including brain CT scan for metastasis and involve an oncologist, and a geriatrician in her care.

I will adjust her treatment, e.g. Risperidone starting dose of 0.5 mg in the evening and titrate up to 2 mg daily while monitoring side effects by performing AIMS.

I will aim for increasing her insight by providing psychoeducation and building a therapeutic relationship by involving her in decision-making.

With her permission I will invite her daughter for a family meeting.

I will focus on increasing her participation in ward activities to minimise her distress from social isolation.

Prior to her discharge, I will involve an OT to assess her level of functioning and a SW for support services at home.

I will screen her for cognitive decline by administering MMSE and frontal lobe testing.

Long-term management

I will focus on maintaining a good therapeutic relationship.

I will continue psychoeducation, monitor mental state, and compliance.

I will identify early warning signs to minimise distress from her psychotic experiences. Social isolation was an important factor in the onset of her illness.

With the help of a SW, I will aim for engaging her in social activities, such as friendship group, etc.

I will communicate with her GP and ask him to monitor her physical health including metabolic parameters. Due to the likelihood of weight gain on atypical antipsychotics, I will monitor her weight and encourage preventative measures such as daily activities and lifestyle modification.

I will explain her that due to a long-term duration of her distress, she will need to take treatment for a few years

Case example 5: OCD

(ID)

Sandra is a seventy-year-old mother of four adults in their 40s, and she lives with her husband. She was interviewed at the outpatient clinic where she sees a local psychiatrist. She gave a long psychiatric history of OCD, anorexia nervosa, and major depression.

(PC)

Sandra presented without symptoms of an acute episode of mental illness.

(PPH)

Sandra's OCD symptoms are the main problems. When unwell, she becomes preoccupied with obsessions of cleanliness and pathological doubt such as checking whether taps are turned off. She wakes up early in the morning to clean the house, vacuums for prolonged periods of time and washes tiles several times.

Her OCD started in childhood with a preoccupation with turning taps off. Initially she attributed her cleanliness to her mother's demands to keep the house clean. She realised that cleaning was an obsession after got married, and the increased amount of time spent on cleaning became problematic. She would vacuum clean under the table while her children were eating. She could not have visitors at home due to urges to clean around them. In addition, she felt an enormous pressure when she was expected to prepare a meal for several people and to have everything ready in a perfect way. She would get up and clean for hours before leaving the house and would feel guilty and agitated, if she did not clean everything according to her expectations. She also used to wash her hands repeatedly, but this was not her main concern. Currently, she has a routine to clean in the mornings before she leaves the house. She also reports religious preoccupation and praying in response to increased anxiety.

Anorexia nervosa started when she was fourteen in response to a critical remark about her appearance. She stated that she did not want to grow up or go to work. She stopped eating, purged, used laxatives, but did not exercise. Her weight dropped from her maximum weight of 45 kg to her minimum weight of 35 kg. She stopped menstruating and experienced pain in her legs. She was admitted to a private clinic.

When she became pregnant, she was less concerned about her eating habits. However, she miscarried and blamed herself for it. She also reported that due to her eating disorder her daughter has epilepsy. When depressed, she becomes more concerned about these guilty beliefs. Her current weight is 40 kg and she is keen to maintain the same weight. She still has residual features of anorexia, such as food restriction. She counts calories and becomes uncomfortable if she loses control over her eating, e.g. after eating ice cream.

She gave a history of many psychiatric admissions in the past, particularly after she overdosed antidepressants in response to low mood and difficulties to cope. She had her first overdose at twenty-three, when her husband was building a garage. When depressed, she becomes fatigued and weak, experiences anhedonia, loss of interest in gardening, suicidal ideation, and thoughts of hopelessness such as 'there is no point'. She becomes overwhelmed by *delusions of pathological guilt* blaming herself for her daughter having epilepsy, son and husband having arthritis, and also for her son's marriage breakdown. She has a history of PND but did not require admission. It is difficult to conclude whether depression precedes or follows a relapse of OCD. Once Sandra becomes overly preoccupied with OCD, she starts cleaning the house at 3 a.m. and depression follows. She was treated with repeated courses of ECT, insulin seizures treatment, and a variety of antidepressants. The most effective were Tranylcypromine with Lithium ten years ago, followed by Fluoxetine with Lithium. Without Lithium, she relapses into severe depression overwhelmed by delusion of guilt.

For the past ten years, she has been treated with Fluoxetine 10 mg twice daily, Quetiapine 25 mg in the evening, Lithium 250 mg in the morning and 125 mg in the evening, and Chlorpromazine 50 mg twice daily. She never had a manic episode, mood incongruent delusions, or perceptual experiences.

(Medical history)

She has a pacemaker but no medication for cardiac arrhythmias. She sees a local cardiologist.

(Relevant personal history)

She was brought up in a strict catholic family. After completing school, she worked as a typist till she married. Her husband has been supportive. She is not close to her family of origin. In spite of long-standing psychiatric history, she managed to bring up four children and keep her marriage. However, she reported that she would not want to go back in her life. Pre-morbidly, she presents as a person with OCPD, preoccupied with morals, routine, cleanliness, and a need for control.

(Family history)

Sandra's niece suffers with OCD and her uncle experienced alcohol dependence.

(Gaps)

I would like to find out more details about OCD symptoms and about a change in her functioning and behaviour when she becomes depressed. I would like to undertake assessment of cognition including frontal lobe screening due to low weight and possible nutritional deficiencies, as well as due to her age. If I had more time, I would ask her how she relates to her catholic upbringing and her religious faith.

Mental State Examination

Sandra presented as an alert and cooperative elderly woman who was well kempt with good eye contact. There was no psychomotor retardation. She had no involuntary movements. She appeared underweight.

Her speech was normal in rate, volume, and prosody.

Her mood was normal.

Her affect was reactive in normal range; at times she became emotional, e.g. when she spoke about her guilt, but she was able to contain her feelings.

There was no formal thought disorder and no current delusions. She denied thoughts of self-harm or harming others. She reported cleaning rituals and other features of OCD (checking and religious preoccupation). In addition, she spoke about anorexia and residual features of the illness. She denied depressive symptoms.

There were no hallucinations.

Her cognition was not formally tested. As judged by responses to questions, it was preserved.

Formulation

Sandra is a seventy-year-old married woman presenting with residual features of mental illness on the background of a long history of OCD, anorexia nervosa and major depression. She is predisposed to all of the above due to strict upbringing and insecure attachment with primary carers. Furthermore, her obsessive compulsive personality makes her vulnerable to develop major depression and anorexia nervosa. She also has a genetic vulnerability for OCD and an affective disorder.

Her eating disorder was triggered by a remark about her appearance. Major depression followed her difficulties to cope with her OCD, in addition to psychosocial stressors. Her need for control is evident in the maintenance of her eating disorder and OCD symptoms.

Diagnoses

Axis I:

1.   Obsessive Compulsive Disorder
2.   Anorexia Nervosa, purging type
3.   Major depressive episode with psychotic features

Differential Diagnosis

Bipolar Affective Disorder II (has increased activity at the time of relapse)

Axis II: Obsessive Compulsive Personality Disorder (need for control, increased morality, rituals, and sense for details)

Axis III: Cardiac arrhythmias, currently pacemaker
Axis IV: Social isolation
Axis V: GAF 60–70 (some mild symptoms and some functional difficulties, but generally functioning pretty well)

Management

Her management will focus on the maintenance of remission and maximizing her functioning.

With her permission, I will speak to her family and obtain collateral information to cover gaps in the history. I will also find out about her past involvement with an Eating Disorder Clinic and suggest a referral.

I will complete cognitive testing including MMSE and frontal lobe tests due to possible nutritional deficits and her age.

I will review investigations available in her file and her previous treatments. Due to the complexity of her past history and treatment, with her permission, I will talk to her previous treating psychiatrist..

I will review her regularly and monitor her mental state for a relapse of depression, OCD and anorexia nervosa, and a risk of self-harm. I will discuss with her about early warning signs as a relapse prevention strategy.

Due to a complexity of diagnoses and a need to identify her early relapse, she will benefit from an ongoing follow-up by a psychiatrist in collaboration with GP.

I will liaise with GP to monitor her weight, metabolic profile, BMD, supplements requirement (due to anorexia nervosa); also to review her trough serum Lithium level, FBC and EUC every three months and TFT every six months.

I will educate her about a risk of Lithium toxicity due to dehydration, if she develops gastrointestinal problems and fever.

With her permission, I will involve her family, especially her husband and find out if there is any functional decline. I will consider involving a clinical psychologist for CBT to modify her thoughts of guilt. I will consider Exposure-Response Prevention for OCD. I will liaise with her cardiologist to be aware of her cardiac condition and its treatment. Her prognosis is guarded due to long-standing illness.

Case example 6: Early Psychosis

(ID)

Helen is a twenty-one-year-old single woman, living with her large extended family of thirteen (parents, older sister, and several uncles and aunties) in their grandparents' own home, now in her third year of university, studying accounting. She regularly attends outpatient clinic for monitoring of her first psychotic episode.

(HPC)

She has been symptom-free over the last seven months on Aripiprazole 5 mg daily.

(PPH)

A year ago she experienced the first psychotic episode. At that time, she presented to hospital with her family with a history of a rapid onset of bizarre thoughts and behaviour, decreased sleep and appetite, and self-neglect. She experienced *persecutory delusions* believing that ghosts spy on her and watch her from the ceilings. She believed that she is the only person who can speak with God (*grandiose delusion*). She expressed *delusions of thoughts insertion* that God puts thoughts into her mind with mystical, metaphysical, and religious content. She also reported *bizarre religious delusions* when she believed that ghosts chose her to give people a message about children and their mothers who died in the water. She also believed that they try to enter her body, but she experienced no pain. She believed that others, especially the ghosts know what she thinks through telepathic means (*delusions of thought broadcasting*) and control her actions (*passivity phenomena*). She also reported (*command auditory hallucinations*) hearing ghosts telling her what to do, e.g. 'wash the dishes' or 'clean the bathroom'. She denied command hallucinations of aggressive nature towards self or others. She reported seeing ghosts (*visual hallucinations*). She could not communicate due to fear of ghosts and she possibly had catatonic features. The only trigger that she could identify was that a month prior to the episode, she was studying for a difficult exam at the university. During this time she had been sleeping poorly, neglecting her food intake, and lost 4 kg in weight.

She was treated with a maximum dose of Aripiprazole 30 mg daily and Lorazepam 4 mg daily. She experienced side effects, stiffness and tremor in the past that responded to a reduction of medication. She was symptom-free after five months of treatment with Aripiprazole.

She reported that she had a brain MRI which was normal. I presume that due to the presence of visual hallucination and the sudden onset of the episode, possibilities of neurological condition like encephalitis was considered.

Prior to this episode, Helen had never been in contact with any mental health services.

She has no forensic history. There is also no significant medical history. She denied any current and past history of illicit drug use. She does not smoke cigarettes.

(Family history)

There is a possible psychiatric history in Helen's maternal aunty in Vietnam, who reportedly was treated in a mental institution.

(Relevant personal history)

Pre-morbidly, she has always been a quiet person, careful and conscientious in her studies, and she likes being with her family. Her early childhood was uneventful. Helen's parents are now fifty-two; both were qualified teachers in Vietnam. Since they migrated to Australia they have been working at a factory as process workers. They have no psychiatric history. She describes herself as belonging to two different cultural groups, which at times conflict with each other.

Migration to Australia brought several challenges into Helen's life. She had to repeat her Year Eleven and Twelve of High School, where she felt older than the other kids. She was not successful in entering university to study psychology and proceeded to study accounting. She described her father as strict and felt significantly pressured by him to succeed academically. She had never been in a relationship. Helen had been in a casual paid employment, prior to her admission to hospital. She was working at a post office sorting out mail mainly over the weekends.

Mental State Examination

She presented as a young woman of Asian background who was wearing casual, clean clothes. She had long dark hair loosely falling on her shoulders. She looked neat and kempt without any evidence of self-neglect. She was pleasant and cooperative in her behaviour and maintained good eye contact. There were no extrapyramidal side effects, akathisia, or tardive dyskinesia.

Her speech was soft, with an ethnic accent. It was normal in rate, volume, and prosody.

Her mood was good and affect was reactive in normal range.

There was no formal thought disorder.

She denied suicidal or homicidal thoughts. She denied current delusions and abnormal perception.

Her cognition was intact.

She had insight into her illness, symptoms, and treatment.

Formulation

Helen is a twenty-one-year-old university student of ethnic background, well-supported by her family. She had one episode of schizophreniform psychosis with initial catatonic features such as mutism a year ago, lasting for five months.

Helen's presentation appears to be in the context of the stress of preparing for a difficult exam. She has a biological vulnerability to mental illness. Developmentally, Helen is at the transition stage between adolescence and adulthood, where she is trying to establish her identity as described by Erikson.

The challenge of her academic performance in accounting has been extremely difficult for Helen, given her interest in psychology and her family's expectation in terms of her education.

The experiences of her family's hardship after migrating to Australia seems to have imposed a sense of responsibility and a desire to satisfy their expectations in terms of her academic achievements. This sense of responsibility may make the time of exams even more difficult for Helen, knowing that any academic failure is likely to cause disappointment.

The issue of Helen's academic achievements will continue to be a significant stressor given her anxious, shy temperament, and the cultural expectations of academic success.

However, Helen has a number of strengths. She is clearly intelligent and articulate. Her conscientiousness and anxious-avoidant personality traits may make her more likely to comply with treatment and to persist with her studies despite her illness.

Diagnosis

Axis I:

Schizophreniform disorder with good prognostic features

Differential Diagnosis

1. Brief psychotic episode (if episode lasted only one month)
2. Schizophrenia (if lasted more than six months)
3. Schizoaffective disorder (if she had a combination of symptoms of mood disorder and schizophrenia, but psychotic symptoms were present for at least two weeks in the absence of mood symptoms. Her presentation did not satisfy this criteria)

Axis II: Nil
Axis III: Nil
Axis IV: Academic pressure during the exam period
          Cultural issues
Axis V: GAF 80–90 (mild anxiety but overall good functioning)

Management

Following the clinical response to Aripiprazole, I will focus on Helen's functional recovery and relapse prevention. I am aware that the relapse rate is high, even in patients like Helen, with good symptomatic and functional recovery, but long-term maintenance treatment with antipsychotics reduces the risk of relapse. I will advice her to take Aripiprazole for a year from the time of remission, provided she remains asymptomatic.

Therapeutic alliance

One of the most important strategies in her management is engagement and the development of a therapeutic alliance. I will work on this therapeutic alliance by ensuring consistency in care, maintenance of confidentiality, and engaging her family in her care. I will include her in making decisions about her treatment. I also ensure that I am available for support and to answer any questions that she has about her illness.

Psychoeducation

I will offer psychoeducation to both her and her family which will facilitate the development of insight in them, and help them better understand her illness and its treatment.

In addition, I will educate them about her medication and its side effects. I will also emphasise the importance of compliance with medication.

I will explain to them that her diagnosis only becomes apparent with time. I will tell them that she had a psychotic episode and give them written information about psychosis. I will emphasize that she was likely to have a biological predisposition for developing mental illness, which could be precipitated by a significant stress. In her case, it was most likely the pressure of the exam driven by her desire for academic achievement. I will discuss the importance of minimising stress and maintaining regular sleep pattern. I will explain that sleep disturbance is a common symptom heralding the onset of a further psychotic episode. As a strategy for relapse prevention, we will discuss about 'early warning signs' of relapse through the exploration of symptoms that she could use to indicate a further episode of psychosis. We will also discuss a management plan that she can initiate, if she starts experiencing the early warning signs. She can monitor her sleep and feelings. She can contact her case worker or the emergency psychiatry team for any advice.

I will provide an individual session for her parents, which can give them a chance to express their personal worries about their daughter. I will invite them for a family education session organized by the team. This will give them an opportunity to ask questions and exchange views with other families with similar experiences.

Other psychological therapies

I will consider her for CBT aiming at reducing relapse rate and improving adherence to medication.

Sociocultural aspects of management

I will liaise with a cultural support worker who can be helpful in my understanding of her cultural beliefs.

Educational support

When Helen could not cope with the pressure of university, she decided to defer her studies for a term. Currently, she is back to studies and coping well. In the future, if required, I will liaise with the university counsellor to facilitate her time off, after she gives me a permission to do so.

Pharmacological treatment

As a consequence of a high dose of Aripiprazole in the past, she experienced side effects, especially sedation and Parkinsonism. These side effects were associated with difficulties to read and concentrate. They significantly diminished after a reduction of her therapeutic dose. Currently, she takes Aripiprazole 5 mg daily and denied that she had any side effects.

Case example 7: Borderline Personality Disorder

(ID)

I saw Alison, a twenty-eight-year-old woman who has been living alone in a rental accommodation since her recent separation from her female partner of two years. She currently works at the local Coles supermarket as an assistant. She was interviewed at the outpatient clinic, where she sees her treating psychiatrist for the treatment of BPD and major depression. She also has a history of poly-substance abuse.

(HPC)

She was discharged form hospital four weeks ago after an eight-week admission with depression. She has been treated with Venlafaxine XR 150 mg in the morning. During the interview, she denied depressive symptoms. She also denied recent suicidal ideation and episodes of self-harm. In addition, she has not been using substances after discharge.

During the recent episode of depression, she was feeling very sad and agitated. She had increased suicidal thoughts and considered gassing herself. She did not sleep, neglected herself, and lost 3 kg in weight. She usually weighs about 50 kg. She was housebound, did not go to work, and was drinking heavily. She heard voices in her head telling her to kill herself and that she was worthless and stupid. She reluctantly agreed with a voluntary admission to hospital. During this time, she remained compliant with her previous antidepressant Escitalopram; however she refused to increase the dose of Escitalopram believing the medication did not work. This episode was precipitated by discovering that her partner of two years, Judi, was having a relationship with one of her female friends. She asked her to leave and ended the relationship two weeks prior to the admission.

(PPH)

Alison has self-harmed from the age of twelve on many occasions, mainly by cutting her forearms superficially, at times requiring stitches. She has been doing this to cope with her mood swings, at times she punishes herself as she believes she is a bad and evil person who deserves punishment. She sometimes burns herself superficially, especially when in conflict with friends or family. She recalled mood swings for as long she as could remember. She describes always feeling sad. This goes back to her primary school years. She reports mood instability and reports her emotional experiences as up and down, and her emotions all over the place. She further says that she snaps very easily and finds her emotional reactions and anger outbursts are out of proportion. She has a poor sense of self and tends to hate herself. She has had thoughts of suicide from the age of twelve. She feels empty and describes her feeling of emptiness as being nothing. She always felt lonely and unloved, and she has chronic low self-esteem.

Self-harm history: She attempted to hang herself at age sixteen about two months after her mother was killed in a MVA. Following this, she was admitted to a psychiatric hospital for about two weeks. She was prescribed Sertraline which she discontinued a week after discharge. She reported no melancholic or psychotic features during this episode, and she could not say if her mood was any different after starting the medication.

Her second hospitalization was precipitated by a break-up with her ex-partner John. She attempted a serious CO poisoning and experienced another depressive episode. She was treated with 6 ECTs and Venlafaxine that she discontinued two weeks after discharge. She described feeling very sad for a few months after this. Diagnosis of BAD was excluded.

(Relevant personal history)

Her father is a fifty-five-year-old man, an alcohol dependent, who lives alone and had no contact with Alison since she was thirteen years old. Her mother died at age forty-one in a MVA. She had chronic depression herself and self-harmed by cutting. Alison said her mother was very critical and she had ambivalent relationship with her. Her parents separated when Alison was thirteen years old due to severe domestic violence. Alison was sexually abused by her paternal grandfather from eighteen till twenty years of age. Alison has two younger stepsisters and one of them also had chronic depression.

From age sixteen to nineteen, she had several brief heterosexual relationships. Many of these men were abusive and had substance abuse disorder. She finds it hard to let anyone close to her and pushes them away in order to prevent them from rejecting her. From age sixteen, she used cannabis, speed, and abused alcohol; she also experimented with cocaine and ecstasy.

She dropped out of school at Year Eleven. From age nineteen to twenty-two, she continued using substances and worked in the sex industry. She stopped cutting and burning but continued using substances. She stopped using all substances by age twenty-four, years after she established a stable relationship with John, age forty-eight, who she met in sex industry. From age twenty-four to twenty-six, she lived with her partner John and used no substances. Self-harm was reduced in frequency and severity. The relationship with John broke down two years later, when she discovered that he was unfaithful to her. She attempted a serious CO poisoning soon after the relationship broke down and had a second hospitalization. She met her current partner, nineteen-year-old Judi in the hospital. Judi also had a diagnosis of BPD. When they lived together, Alison gave up substances and started working at the Coles supermarket again.

There is no significant medical or forensic history.

(Functional impact of the illness)

Of note is Alison's emotional instability and difficulties to cope with stress that cause repeated self-harm and use of substances to relieve emotional trauma. Her low self-esteem predisposes her to a poor choice of partner with further implications on her self-esteem.

(Risks)

Due to emotional instability and repeated depressive episodes, she remains at a long-term risk of self-harm that can turn into a suicidal attempt when she faces major life crises such as losses.

(Gaps)

I would like to obtain more details about her interpersonal functioning and social activities. I would also find out what she sees as an outcome of her treatment and whether she would like to engage in psychological treatment.

Mental State Examination

Alison presented as a young and slim woman of Caucasian background, wearing a white shirt and jeans. She was clean and kempt. Her blond hair was loosely falling on her shoulders.

She was calm and cooperative during the interview. Rapport was easily established. There were no involuntary movement.

Her speech was normal in rate, volume, and prosody. She spoke spontaneously.

Her mood was improved.

Her affect was euthymic. It was congruent with her mood and thoughts.

There was no formal thought disorder.

There were no delusions, no suicidal or homicidal ideation, and no negative cognitions.

Her insight was partial, she reported compliance with Venlafaxine XR for a depressive episode. She was aware that her self-harm was a response to stress but she was not aware of features of her personality.

Formulation

Alison is a twenty-eight-year-old woman with a recent episode of major depression on the background of BPD and a past history of poly-substance abuse, currently in a stable mental state.
She has a biological vulnerability to develop depressive illness with a history of depression in her mother and stepsister. Her insecure attachment with mother and the early loss of her mother in adolescent age, as well as the sexual abuse by her grandfather, predispose her to personality disorder and depression. It is possible that the early losses may have led to dysfunctional assumptions about self with a tendency to self-blame and self criticality, leading further to difficulties in negotiating the early challenges of childhood and adolescence. As a consequence, she uses unhealthy coping strategies to deal with stressors such as self-harming behaviour and substance use. These would have then

impacted on forming peer group relationships. Psychologically, she is stagnated at the Erikson's stage of role confusion.

Losses of close relationships and a fear of abandonment were important precipitants of her depressive episodes. Her recent depressive episode seemed to be also in the context of a relationship stress. Alcohol abuse was an additional precipitant.

Fortunately, she has positive prognostic factors which include her ability to engage in treatment and financial independence provided by ongoing employment. She also has a good response to treatment with antidepressants and denies recent substance use.

Differential diagnosis

Axis I:
Major depressive episode moderate to severe, in remission
Dysthymic disorder, early onset
Grief reaction
Poly-substance abuse
Axis II: Borderline personality disorder
Axis III: Nil
Axis IV: Recent relationship break-up
Axis V: GAF 50–60 (moderate symptoms and difficulties in functioning)

Management

As her depression is currently in remission, I will focus on her BPD and on improving her coping strategies, as I am aware that the presence of BPD is a predictor of accelerated relapse after remission from a major depressive episode. In addition, treatment of BPD also has a good impact on the management of depression (but treatment of depression does not result in remission of BPD).

I will complete her assessment and obtain collateral information that can help me decide about the most suitable psychological therapy for her. I will discuss options of different types of therapy with her and come to a join decision.

She can be suitable for DBT as she has a history of suicidal and self-harming behaviour and also has a history of emotional instability and interpersonal difficulties. (The standard length of DBT is approximately one year). It involves one hour of individual therapy per week, more than two hours of group skill training per week (for either six or twelve months), along with a requirement for all therapists in the program to meet weekly as a group.

She can also benefit from MBT (Mentalisation-based therapy) which has effect on both depression and BPD, and it is as efficacious as DBT. The principles of MBT can be used in everyday practice. The principles of MBT have lot of in common with Gubderson's 'good enough' treatment for BPD. The therapy will help her reflect on her own state of mind, which she usually inhibits because of early trauma and abuse.

She would also be suitable for psychodynamic therapy based on the Kohut model of self-psychology. Psychodynamic therapy can help her identify important unconscious patterns that are not available to her, with an intention to increase her affect tolerance, delay impulsive actions, and provide insight into relationship problems.

I will encourage her compliance with medication due to past episodes of depression, serious past suicidal attempts, and non-compliance with treatment. For his purpose, I will use psychoeducation to increase awareness about her illness, treatment, and possible side effects. Venlafaxine can have an additional benefit for symptoms of affective dysregulation and impulsivity of BPD.

During the outpatient reviews, I will monitor her mental state and identify early signs of relapse. I will aim for an outpatient treatment. If a hospital admission is required in crisis, this should be brief unless she has another affective episode.

I will monitor her for substance abuse. If required, I will use Motivation Interview principles to encourage abstinence from substances. Depending on her need, I will offer her an involvement of D&A team.

Due to her past sexual history and a history of drug use, with her consent, I will screen her for STD including HIV, syphilis, and hepatitis C.

I will provide her with emergency numbers and contacts at the crisis team after hours.

GOOD LUCK!

Abbreviations

AIMS—Abnormal involuntary movement scale
AN—Anorexia nervosa
ANA—Antinuclear antibody
ASPD—Antisocial personality disorder
ARAFMI—Association of relatives and friends of the mentally ill
AVO—Apprehended violence order
BMI—Body mass index
BMD—Bone Marrow Density
BN—Bulimia nervosa
BAD I—Bipolar affective disorder I
BAD II—Bipolar affective disorder II
BPD—Borderline personality disorder
BSL—Blood sugar level
CBT—Cognitive behavioural therapy
CCM—Community case manager
CPG—Clinical practice guidelines
CVA—Cerebrovascular accident
CXR—Chest x-ray
D&A—Drug and alcohol
DSH—Deliberate self-harm
DSP—Disability support pension
ED—Eating disorder
EE—Expressed emotions
EUC—Electrolyte urea creatinine
EWS—Early warning signs
FI—Family intervention
FBC—Full blood count
GGT—Gamma-glutamyl transferase
HPC—History of presenting complains
HTN—Hypertension
ID—Identifying data
IHD—Ischaemic heart disease
IPT—Interpersonal psychotherapy
IVD—Intravenous drug
LFT—Liver function test
MAOI—Monoamine oxidase inhibitor
MCV—Mean cell volume

MDT—Multidisciplinary team
MI—Motivational interview
MOYB—Month of the year backwards
MS—Multiple sclerosis
MSU—Midstream urine
NGO—National government organisation
NICE—National institute of clinical excellence
OCD—Obsessive-Compulsive disorder
OCPD—Obsessive-Compulsive personality disorder
OT—Occupational therapist
PC—Presenting complaints
PE—Pulmonary embolism
PND—Postnatal depression
PPH—Past psychiatric history
SLE—Systemic lupus erythematosis
SOL—Space occupying lesion
SNRI—Serotonin-norepinephrine reuptake inhibitor
SSRI—Serotonin selective reuptake inhibitor
STM—Short-term memory
SW—Social worker
T3—Triiodothyronine
TBI—Traumatic brain injury
TB—Thought broadcast
TCA—Tricyclic antidepressant
TD—Tardive dyskinesia
TI—Thought insertion
TLE—Temporal lobe epilepsy
TOC—Treatment of choice
TRD—Treatment resistant depression
TW—Thought withdrawal
UDS—Urine drug screen
WCC—White cell cont

Recommended Reading

Andreasen N.C. Thought, Language, and Communication Disorders. *Arch Gen Psychiatry* 1979; 36:1315–21

Australian and New Zealand Journal of Psychiatry

Australasian Psychiatry

CPG (College Practice Guidelines) RANZCP

DSM—IV—TR

Fish's clinical psychopathology (third edition)

Gabbard, Psychodynamic Psychiatry in Clinical Practice

Kaplan and Sadock's Synopsis of Psychiatry

NICE Guidelines: *www.nice.org.uk*

OCI Kaveh notes

RANZCP web site: *http://www.ranzcp.org/*

The Maudsley Prescribing Guidelines

Stahl, Essential Psychopharmacology

www.anzapt.org

www.ingramcontent.com/pod-product-compliance
Lightning Source LLC
Chambersburg PA
CBHW022014170526
45157CB00003B/1247